VISCERAL MANIPULATION II

Visceral Manipulation II

Jean-Pierre Barral

ILLUSTRATIONS BY
Jacques Roth

Eastland Press
SEATTLE

Originally published as *Manipulations viscerales (II)*
Maloine (Paris), 1987.

English language edition © 1989 by Eastland Press, Incorporated
P.O. Box 12689, Seattle, Washington, 98111
All rights reserved.

Library of Congress Catalog Card Number: 87-82743
International Standard Book Number: 0-939616-09-2
Printed in the United States of America.

Edited by Denise Gilles (French edition), Stephen Anderson, Ph.D.
& Daniel Bensky, D.O. (English edition).
Book design by Catherine L. Nelson.
Photolithoprinted by Cushing-Malloy, Incorporated,
Ann Arbor, Michigan, 1989.

Second printing, 1994

Table of Contents

Chapter One:
Introduction

Table of Contents

Introduction

I will presume at the outset that the reader is familiar with the earlier book *(Visceral Manipulation)* by myself and P. Mercier, and will therefore not explain in detail the essential concepts of mobility, motility, listening, induction, etc. I would, however, like to clarify several aspects of the osteopathic visceral concept and its applications, including the treatment of children. In this first chapter I will also describe a variety of clinical tests and recent findings of interest.

Lesional Chains

As stated by Rollin Becker, D.O., and repeated by me many times, "Only the tissues know." It is not uncommon for tissues to lose their normal functions, including their contractile, elastic and distensible properties. When the structure of these tissues is modified, an area of stronger mechanical tension is created which I refer to as a restriction. In osteopathic parlance this phenomenon is also known as a lesion. A restriction has a detrimental effect on all neighboring structures, and affects the axes of motion of organs, as well as the directions of force lines in the body. As an experienced practitioner can feel, restrictions may literally attract the hand. These tissue restrictions are the beginning of *lesional chains*.

An injured tissue does not remain isolated. Because of an imbalance of its environmental mechanical tensions, the organ's attachments lose their usual distensibility and give rise to a membranous restriction or lesion. This may result from direct or indirect trauma, or secondarily from an inflammatory illness. For example, during and especially after viral hepatitis, Glisson's capsule and the suspensory ligament of the liver lose their normal elasticity.

Pressure, mobility, motility and other forces are poorly transmitted through a restriction, with resulting disturbance of the balance of both local and whole-body membrane systems. This distorted reciprocal tension causes peritoneal/visceral articulation problems and internal organ dysfunctions.

A tissue or membrane which has lost its elasticity contributes to the creation of a general mechanical problem where normally one would find an orderly process. This is the lesional chain where one link disturbs another, and so on, until a symptom appears. Such imbalances take place in stages, following the laws of compensation and adaptation associated with the body's perpetual state of change. As long as compensation is possible, the progression of the problem is imperceptible. It is when all the adaptive processes have been exhausted that the symptom suddenly appears. Sometimes this happens with a speed and severity disproportionate to the most recent provocation; an example is acute low back pain which develops during a seemingly ordinary movement. Because of the lesional chain process, a symptom can appear at a site distant from the primary lesion.

One can try to trace this chain by going from the symptom to the cause. But be wary of intellectual exercises which provide a neat, connected explanation for everything. It would not be helpful to trace a lesional chain from the fifth metatarsal to the sella turcica by many different routes, each more logical and attractive than the last. It would be better for you and your patient if you followed with careful palpation and listened to the tissues instead of getting carried away by memorized theoretical strategies.

Excretion/Secretion

Interestingly, my best results have been obtained on those organs which have an excretory canal or at least an emptying system. Using fluoroscopy, we have been able to see the effects of visceral manipulation on the gallbladder, common bile duct, pylorus, bladder, and uterine tubes. On the other hand, we have never been able to convincingly demonstrate its efficacy on organs lacking excretory canals, such as the spleen.

All excretory canals need to retain good longitudinal axial extension in order to perform their functions properly. These canals, which include the duodenum, common bile duct and ureter, have a variety of shapes and diameters. We have found that the best way to improve the emptying ability of a tube is to stretch it along its longitudinal axis. In general this means anchoring the proximal part while pushing the distal part even more distally along the axis, or vice versa. Clinical experience has often confirmed transit improvement in, for example, the common bile duct and pylorus.

We performed experiments in 1980 with the common bile duct, in which stretching appeared to increase the evacuation of bile. The only published data of a similar nature that I know of involved the ureter, whose efficiency was increased 40% by stretching *(Scali & Giraud, 1986)*.

Pressures

In the human body, different pressures, which originate from the pulmonary system, confront and harmonize with each other *(Visceral Manipulation, pp. 15-16)*. The membranes of the body transmit and integrate the different pressures. The redistribution of pressures takes place via transversely-oriented structures such as the diaphragm, thoracic inlet and pelvic inlet, as well as via longitudinally-oriented ligamentous structures such as those interconnecting the diaphragm, liver, intestines, stomach, etc. These transmitters and shock-absorbers can only fulfill their roles when they have adequate elasticity and distensibility. Fibrosis and sclerosis cause problems in the distribution of pressures and contribute to the disruption of visceral cohesion.

Reported values for these pressures vary little regardless of the source of information. Averages for various areas of the body are:

- skull: $+15\,cm\ H_2O$
- thorax: $-5\,cm\ H_2O$
- upper abdomen: $+5\,cm\ H_2O$
- middle abdomen: $+15\,cm\ H_2O$
- lower abdomen: $+20\,cm\ H_2O$
- pelvis: $+30\,cm\ H_2O$

An abnormality in these pressures disturbs an organ's excretions and, I believe, its secretions as well. Coughing produces pressures of $+100\,cm\ H_2O$ in the bladder, and hard pushing for defecation can bring the intrarectal pressure up to $+200$ instead of the normal $+50\,cm\ H_2O$. The body can only support these high pressures briefly.

Increased pressure in the intestine increases the likelihood of diverticulosis. Chronic increases of abdominal pressure may lead to development of hiatal hernias, inguinal hernias, varicose veins and hemorrhoids. The latter are partly due to increases of abdominal and portal vein pressure.

Reflexogenic Zones

These are zones that demonstrate the greatest reaction to visceral techniques because of their dense innervation. Included within this group are the junction zones between the different parts of the digestive tract and their visceral attachments, i.e., mesenteries, ligaments and omenta.

We observed early in our studies that manipulation of certain junction zones has a rapid and general effect on spasms and visceral pain and, in addition, rapidly affects the digestive system. I refer to such areas as "sphincter-like junctions." Although not everyone accepts this concept, I believe that it is valid, particularly for the pylorus. It is true that this junction is almost permanently open, a fact that we have verified using endoscopy. Nonetheless, it is surrounded by circular muscle fibers which, when in spasm, can be felt by palpation. The pylorus also has the distinctive ability to move laterally from one side of the midline to the other during peristalsis, due to a combination of rotational and transverse contractions. This increases the efficiency of gastroduodenal transit.

Such highly reflexogenic zones affect each other strongly. Eating, for example, stimulates intestinal functions via the gastrocolic reflex. As another example, spasms of the duodenojejunal flexure can be treated by manipulating the ileocecal junction. In terms of general treatment, one must utilize these zones to involve the entire visceral system and to enhance the body's response to treatment. In general, when you want to treat a sphincter-like junction, you should work on the sphincter immediately below it. For example, manipulation of the pylorus affects the lower esophageal sphincter (gastro-esophageal junction).

At the end of a treatment session, check to see that the sphincter-like zones affecting the areas you worked on (e.g., the sphincter of Oddi and the duodenojejunal flexure) are open and moving synchronously. It is also a good idea to check more proximally and distally (e.g., pylorus and ileocecal valve). This is done by either motility testing or local listening. The following are, in my experience, the most effective sphincter-like junctions:

- gastroesophageal junction and gastric cardia
- pylorus
- sphincter of Oddi
- duodenojejunal flexure
- ileocecal junction
- rectal area

Over the course of many years of palpating abdomens we have discovered certain common "critical zones." I consider them critical because when they are tight or in spasm the functioning of the body is significantly impaired. Of particular interest are the gallbladder, sphincter of Oddi, and ileocecal junction. These are frequent "targets" for somatization of stress, i.e., environmental stressors are particularly likely to produce irritation and spasm in these critical zones. For some reason the mind likes to use the sphincters as an outlet. If I were forced to choose only two areas to work on to release a patient's abdomen, I would, without hesitation, choose the sphincter of Oddi and the ileocecal junction. They should always be stretched; freeing them creates a general relaxation whereby digestion and abdominal circulation are improved.

The peritoneal attachments also have powerful reflexogenic possibilities. For example, concentrating your manipulation on the roots of the mesentery or sigmoid mesocolon will result in a response from the associated organs. The parietal peritoneum has a sensitive innervation which should be utilized as much as possible. The ligaments and mesenteric roots are the best intermediaries for obtaining a quick release of the peritoneum in general. Use the techniques described in chapter 2, p. 45 for optimal results.

Diagnostic Tests and Methods

In *Visceral Manipulation* we discussed mobility and motility tests. I will now describe other tests which facilitate general and local diagnosis. I would like to emphasize that when performing these tests you should always approach patients consistently from the same side. Generally speaking, right-handed practitioners should position themselves on the right side of the patient. The use of topographical anatomy in visceral manipulation necessitates precise reference marks. Changing sides modifies your orientation and your perspective of the organs, which can lead to errors and make your treatment less effective.

GENERAL LISTENING

Osteopathic diagnosis involves using the hands to "listen" to the patient's body. When a particular tissue is ill, it loses its elasticity, disrupts the patient's membranous equilibrium, and becomes a new axis or pivot point for the motions of mobility and motility. On palpation, as you concentrate on the motion of the tissues, you will feel your hands being drawn to dysfunctional areas because they move much less than do the healthy tissues. This is the same phenomenon you experience when you touch an abdomen which has a scar: you quickly feel your hand being drawn to the scar because it is much more tense and rigid than the surrounding tissues.

When performing listening (either general or local) it is vitally important that you be as passive and accepting as possible. Be careful not to project yourself onto the patient. One way to accomplish the proper mindset is to imagine that the hand you are listening with is attracting or absorbing the body rather than extending your sense of touch through the person's body (which is done to feel for motility as well as to perform cranial osteopathy). Another helpful hint is to inhale while you are listening; this makes it easier to be passive and to focus on the attraction between your hand and the body. Conversely, while extending your sense of touch it helps to exhale. One final hint: when listening, pay attention to the first motion that you feel because that is the correct response.

For example, if the liver is very tense and heavy (as is the case in hepatitis) it will attract the right pleura, the right lung, the attachments of the lung to the right cervical vertebrae, and the head. By listening from the head, as described below, you will be able to feel this attraction immediately and pinpoint its origin.

General listening consists simply of placing your hands on the patient in such a way that you can collect information about the entire body. By doing this you can feel where the major areas of restriction are. The hands are passive and searching for soft tissue tensions. In order for the information to be reliably transmitted, the patient's body must be somewhat precariously balanced so that it will move in response to a small amount of force. I recommend doing the test with the patient in either the standing or seated position; when the body is supine it is supported at too many points. However, one problem with the standing position is that it is usually more difficult for the practitioner (particularly short practitioners working on tall patients).

In the seated position *(Illustration 1-1)*, the patient sits with his legs hanging down from the examining table and the practitioner standing behind him. Place one hand flat on the posterior parietal region of the skull, either along the axis of the vertebral column, or perpendicular to it. The other hand either remains free or is placed under the coccyx; if the latter, that forearm is oriented along the spine.

The patient's body will spontaneously direct itself toward the restriction; slight pressure from your hand will reveal and slow down the movement. The patient must be passive; unfortunately, your request that he remain passive will sometimes cause him to unintentionally contract some part of the body, distorting your perceptions and interfering with the process of listening. The purpose of this exercise is to feel a relatively stronger muscular/membranous tension which very subtly pulls the body toward it. Therefore, it is sometimes better to subtly encourage or amplify the movement of the body toward the restriction in order to overcome these slight, unintentional contractions. This is a motion on the order of motility, not mobility; i.e., the amount of force you use to start and follow this procedure through is similar to that used for induction, and much less than that used for mobilization. You can always check your findings by repeating the procedure with your other hand on the head; if you are truly feeling the correct motion, it will feel the same with either hand. If you are projecting your own belief onto the patient's body, it will usually feel differently depending on which hand you are using. With a little experience, you can easily overcome this difficult starting point.

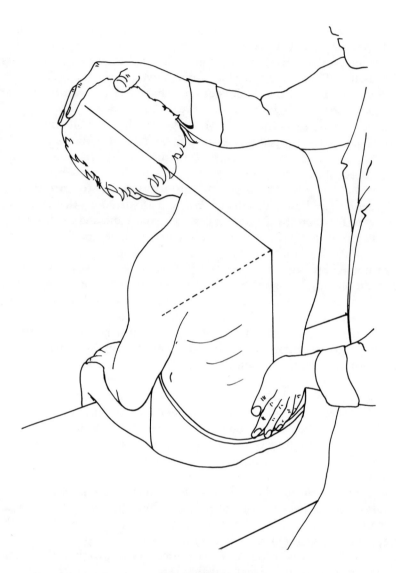

Illustration 1-1
General Listening: Diagnostic Angle

Diagnostic Angle

Suppose that the patient is bending forward; this would indicate an anterior problem. The more that the patient is bending forward, the lower you would look to find the problem. If his forward bending is accompanied by a sidebending to the left, the restriction will be situated on the left, and the extent of bending to the left will indicate the distance of the restriction from the midline. The combination of these two bending motions will enable you to locate the restriction rather precisely. That is, the bending motions will form an angle, the apex of which will be situated at the site of the restriction. The apex can be found by using the angle between the cervical spine and thoracolumbar spine, the cervicothoracic and lumbar spine, the entire spine and the table top, etc. There are many possibilities.

This technique is very useful because it enables you to rapidly locate the pathological region without having to search for it point by point. I want to emphasize that this method is useful to find any pathological area, not just those involving the viscera. One can also use it for articular pathologies. In this manner, an injury to R7 gives rise to an angle formed by the thoracic and lumbar spines, the apex of which will be found on the seventh costovertebral articulation.

LOCAL DIFFERENTIAL DIAGNOSIS

This approach consists of using local listening in order to precisely locate the injured attachment or organ. Please note that here I am using the word "listening" in a slightly different sense than in *Visceral Manipulation*. In that book we used the term to describe what you do to detect motility, which is an ongoing process; here the term "local listening" is used to describe how you feel the state of the body or a particular organ. The main difference is actually in the thought process involved with the procedure. For local listening, the hand passively receives information from the neighboring tissues. You do *not* try to extend your sense of touch through your hand; rather you passively attract the body up through your hand. This difference is crucial because if you extend your touch through your hand you will be picking up motility or the craniosacral rhythm, rather than doing local listening. While you are listening, it often helps to breathe in, as this makes it easier to be accepting and passive. Pay attention only to what you feel in the heel and palm of your hand, not the fingers. And again, focus on what you first feel, as this is the correct perception.

To listen to the abdomen, have the patient lie supine and place your more sensitive hand on the midline with the heel just above the umbilicus and the fingertips below the xiphoid process. Right-handed practitioners usually use the right hand and therefore sit or stand on the right side of the patient. When a particular tissue is too tense, it attracts the hand. You will actually feel the hand move toward the restriction. This is often a step-by-step process. For example, with your hand on the midline you may feel the heel of your hand move toward the right costal margin. You should follow this motion until it cannot move any farther, perhaps to a point 2 cm to the right and 2 cm superior to the umbilicus. Then reposition your hand so that it is placed parallel to the midline with the heel at that point, and repeat the procedure until there is no more movement. If there is no significant restriction in the trunk, your hand will not be attracted to any particular place during local listening; nor should you feel attraction when rechecking following a treatment.

Local listening can also be applied to a specific organ or tissue. Describing this will clarify the difference between local listening and listening to motility. For example, to listen to the motility of the kidney, place your thenar or hypothenar eminence over the surface projection of the organ, then push slightly posterior and extend your sense of touch until you can feel the alternating external and internal rotation of the organ *(Visceral Manipulation, p. 198)*. If there is no problem, both phases of motility will have good amplitude and a smooth quality. Thus, listening to motility tunes you in to the ongoing process of the organ's inherent motion. Local listening of the kidney is quite different, however. Placing your hand in the same position, you attract the kidney, listening for just one motion. In general, and to oversimplify: if there is no problem, you will feel nothing; if there is a second degree ptosis, you will feel an external rotation; if there is a third degree ptosis, you will feel an internal rotation. (For more detail, see chapter 9, p. 213.) Local listening therefore enables you to check the state of the tissues.

Inhibition points (see below) are very useful when combined with local listening. To continue with the example given above, your hand has moved toward the right upper quadrant of the abdomen, which contains many structures such as the liver, ascending colon, and hepatic flexure. If you think that the movement you are feeling upon local listening is pulling your hand toward the hepatic flexure, inhibit that structure by applying a gentle pressure just below the lateral aspect of the costal margin. If the hand is no longer attracted in that direction, you may conclude that there is a restriction of this flexure. The complete procedure, therefore, consists of using an inhibition point to confirm the location of a restriction. If the attraction of the hand is negated, this confirms that there is a restriction of that structure.

When a problem is present, after determining which organ is involved, you then assess the motility of that organ to further refine your diagnosis. For example, if the liver has no motility at all, it means that the patient has a severe, general energy problem (usually with a large psychological component); restriction of the liver in inspir (meaning that it goes into inspir, but not into expir) indicates a history of inflammation such as hepatitis; and restriction of the liver in expir indicates a problem of bile evacuation. In fact, this is the general concept of organ restriction: when an organ is restricted in inspir it is primarily a problem of the organ itself; when it is restricted in expir it is primarily a problem of fluid evacuation.

I have checked my diagnoses numerous times in order to confirm the value of local differential diagnosis by examining patients suffering from various well-documented illnesses such as hepatitis, peptic ulcer, and renal lithiasis. You can test your own ability by trying to find a surgical scar on a patient who is dressed. In addition, you should practice with colleagues using artificial restrictions. For example, have the colleague create a "restriction" of a patient's right knee with hand pressure and try to discover which knee is involved by placing your hands on the patient's abdomen. Repeat this procedure about ten times (obviously with your eyes shut). It is necessary to constantly practice in order to acquire palpatory skills which are reproducible, and to gain confidence. I repeat that the hands are the osteopath's only tool. You should train them and continually develop their sensitivity. It is wise to recheck your ability at periodic intervals.

Inhibition Points

An injured tissue draws the body and your hand toward it. However, by gently pressing against the tissue you can inhibit its effect on the rest of the body. I believe that this inhibition is due to a mechanical effect on the continuity of the fibers, but have no proof of this. In any case, this effect is easily demonstrated clinically. Do not press too hard or you will reinforce the attracting tension. For example, if on general listening you feel a pull toward the right hypochondrium, place the fingers of one hand under the liver to push it very slightly posterosuperiorly, keeping the other hand in the general listening position. If the body is no longer bent forward and to the right, this would strongly tend to confirm the presence of a hepatic problem. If, on the other hand, the position is retained, a rib restriction is probable. You could also inhibit the rib restriction by exerting a slight pressure on the transverse process which articulates with the rib. A halt or modification in the movement would signify a restriction of that rib.

Try this technique yourself and you will be surprised by both its speed and its wide applicability. As always, it is best to follow the tissues, for they are better guides than your own reasoning. While using inhibition points will allow you to pinpoint the main organ that is involved in a problem, this does not necessarily mean that the problem is primarily a mechanical one. For example, liver involvement could be due to the use of birth control pills, hepatitis, etc., and not necessarily to ligamentous restrictions. If the birth control pills are the problem, visceral manipulation will have no lasting effect.

One method of corroborating the results of general listening is accomplished with the patient in the supine position. Using both hands, plantar flex the feet, maintain the flexion and then release the pressure without taking your hands off the feet. The foot which dorsiflexes itself faster will be on the same side as the most important restriction. To assume accuracy, you should apply quite a bit of flexion. You can also perform this test simply by listening. Place both hands on the superior surfaces of the feet. The foot which seems to dorsiflex is on the injured side *(Illustration 1-2)*. This will not be a strong movement, but rather an intention of a movement which is very distinctly perceived with practice.

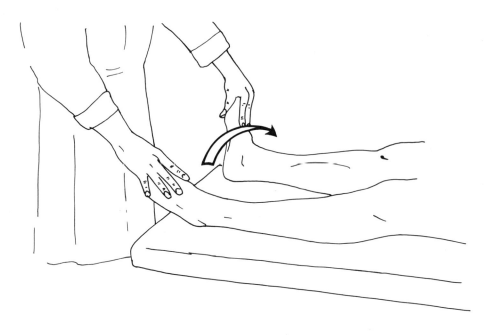

Illustration 1-2
Listening: Lower Limbs

Listening through the feet is extremely important because many people have significant lower extremity restrictions. Consider a patient who, upon general listening, bends far forward anteriorly and rotates to the right in the standing position. From this test alone it is extremely difficult to differentiate between right lower quadrant abdominal problems and those of the right lower extremity. When the patient sits down, the lower extremities relax and lose their effect on the rest of the body. Therefore, if the patient sits down and the results of general listening remain the same, you can be sure that the restriction is in fact an abdominal one. However, if the results of general listening change dramatically or even become normal, the significant restriction is likely to be in the right lower extremity. Use of the ankle flexion test and inhibition points on the lower extremity (ankle, knee, etc.) will enable you to pinpoint the location of the restriction.

To test the sensitivity of my students I create an artificial restriction: I gently pinch the patient's skin or muscle without the student seeing it, and then ask the student to locate the affected area. Students who are accustomed to this exercise perform it without error. I would like to remind skeptics that all the senses, including touch, can be trained to a high level of acuity. The ability of a wine taster to use the power of his senses to identify a bottle of wine to its appropriate time and place is not commonly contested; is this not much more subtle and challenging than the skills I am discussing here?

What you find on general listening is just the area of the body that requires treatment at that time. It is not necessarily a "key lesion" that is written in stone. I usually repeat general listening after each phase of treatment or after working on the indicated area. In these circumstances, the general listening will often change during the course of the session. For example, you may first feel the stomach and later the right kidney. This is normal and you should only treat what you find. Do not focus on more than three organs during one session. This is more than the body can take and you can create new restrictions. When I say "focus on" I am not implying that you should only touch two or three organs, but rather that you should only treat that number. Naturally, you can and should work on their attachments to other organs. For example, to work on the right kidney it is necessary to work on its attachments with the liver, ascending colon and cecum, but I would still consider this as treating one organ only.

THE ADSON-WRIGHT TEST

The Adson-Wright (also known as Sotto-Hall) test consists of palpating the patient's radial pulse in the seated position while taking that arm into external rotation and abduction. At the end of the movement, the patient is asked to rotate his head first to one side and then the other. During this movement the pulse should remain constant in intensity and frequency. The test is positive when the pulse is diminished or suppressed, a phenomenon attributed to compression of the subclavian artery. This artery, with the brachial plexus, goes through the "inter-scalene passage," which is bounded at the front by the anterior scalene muscle and at the back by the middle and posterior scalenes *(Illustration 1-3)*. If there is a thick pleural ligament or a minor scalene muscle (only occasionally present) between the plexus and the artery, and if the angle at which R1 comes off the vertebra is particularly oblique, the passage closes up. The plexus and the artery are already close together in women, in whom R1 usually comes off more obliquely than in men. We have also obtained positive results in cases involving extra ribs or enlarged cervical transverse processes. Problems such as radicular pain or circulatory disturbances occur where there is compression.

When the patient holds the position of abduction and external rotation of the arm, the passage shrinks and the patient feels a sensation of heavy or "dead" fingers. He then wriggles his fingers and moves his arm to activate circulation. When this type of paresthesia occurs upon awakening, it may be accompanied by headaches which stop within several hours. These phenomena are caused by certain sleeping positions, e.g., lying on

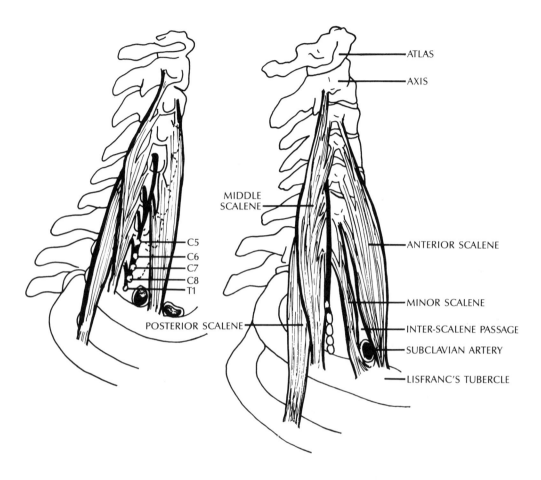

Illustration 1-3
Inter-scalene Passage (after Lazortes)

the stomach with the head on the forearms, or in the supine position with the hands behind the back of the neck. In such cases, sleep does not perform its usual healing function and is often interrupted by nightmares. The patient cannot remain for prolonged periods of time with arms raised or head tilted back. Fifteen years ago, operations were often performed on such patients (usually without success).

I use the Adson-Wright test in my osteopathic practice, and am surprised by how often I obtain positive results. After thousands of cases, I realized that the test was positive on the side of the restriction whether the restriction was of articular or visceral origin. When the pulse diminishes with 30° of external rotation or less, the problem is usually related to the mechanics of the thoracic outlet. When it diminishes with 30 to 90° of rotation, it is often due to a visceral restriction. If it only diminishes when the patient turns his head, it is usually due to a mechanical restriction of the upper thoracic or cervical region. However, I occasionally take the precaution of obtaining X-rays to eliminate the possibility of any skeletal abnormalities.

My colleague Louis Rommeveaux, D.O. (who also teaches at the European School of Osteopathy in Maidstone, U.K. and Le College International d'Osteopathie in France) and I selected several patients who presented positive Adson-Wright test results to undergo experiments using the Doppler device, which makes it possible to look objectively at arterial blood circulation. We performed these studies in 1982 with the help of Dr. Morzol of Grenoble, France, and chose to examine the radial and vertebral/basilar arteries. We first recorded the objective results of the Adson-Wright test and then treated the patients with cranial, articular and visceral manipulation techniques. The visceral manipulations gave best results when the forces used were so minimal as to be incapable of restoring arterial circulation by themselves. We also carried out several placebo manipulations which had no effect. Doppler testing showed, without any doubt, that improvement or restoration of blood flow was possible, but there was no explanation for the mechanism. How can a slight manipulation of an abdominal organ immediately restore arterial circulation to the head or arm?

My theory is that the effect involves the parietal peritoneum as intermediary. The peritoneum receives certain sensory fibers arising from the phrenic nerve, which interconnects with the subclavian nerve. Abnormal stimulation of these nerves can cause contraction of the subclavius muscle and vasoconstriction of the subclavian artery. By freeing these tissues, one can release these abnormal effects. The inter-scalene passage, no longer shrunken by the contraction of the subclavius muscle, regains its normal depth and the artery assumes its normal tone.

I am aware that this is merely speculation, and encourage other researchers to share their conclusions with us. I am certain of one thing: that the speed of the arterial response can only be explained by a reflex effect. The spasms mentioned above are surely pathological for the passages, which are already anatomically narrow. My conclusion from this study is that a positive Adson-Wright test indicates the side of the restriction. An ipsilateral restriction is often of visceral reflex origin. Only very slight forces are needed for visceral manipulation when you are precise.

To complete the Adson-Wright technique, continue taking the radial pulse with one hand, and with the other hand create inhibition points and note subsequent changes. For example, let's say you obtain an Adson-Wright test result which is positive on the right, and general listening implicates the liver. Very gently push the liver posterosuperiorly (Illustration 1-4). If the pulse comes back, you should consider a hepatic problem. (Later we shall see how to refine this diagnosis.) If the Adson-Wright test is still positive (i.e., the pulse does not come back), try inhibition points on other locations until you find the causal restriction.

As another example, assume your vertebral motility tests have indicated a transverse process restriction at C5/C6. You can apply an inhibition point here, note subsequent effects on the Adson-Wright test, and so on. An inhibition point which liberates subclavian arterial flow indicates the area of the restriction, which you can then pinpoint by local differential diagnosis, as explained above.

BLOOD PRESSURE

In osteopathy, blood pressure should be recorded in a consistent manner; I take the blood pressure in both arms. In a young patient, the values are normally equal. If there is a difference in systolic pressure of more than 10mm Hg between the two sides, the one with the lower value is the site of a restriction. This conclusion is based on my

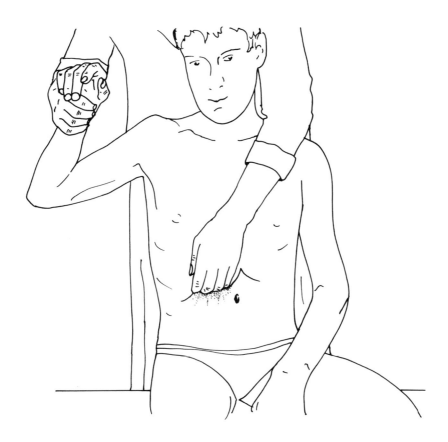

Illustration 1-4
Completed Adson-Wright Test

observations of several thousand cases. In older patients, where arteries may differ in hardness, a difference must be more than 15 mm Hg to be considered significant. This difference is not commonly utilized in conventional medicine, in which it is attributed to a few rare cases of arterial coarctation (stricture) and to problems of the fibrous arterial sheath. Compression of the aortic isthmus is thought to be demonstrated by arterial hypertension of the upper limbs, contrasting with arterial hypotension of the lower limbs.

I believe that the difference in systolic pressure is related to pathology of soft tissues. As with the Adson-Wright test, it can be explained by a phrenic or vagal reflex action, or a fibrous injury to the inter-scalene passage or various associated ligaments. With other important injuries, both the Adson-Wright test and arterial pressure are affected. It is easy to take arterial pressure and to feel a radial pulse. A positive (i.e., abnormal) result from either test is enough to tell me that something is amiss. Proper manipulation should normalize these values. These are two of the few objective tests available for evaluating the effects of manipulation.

If the test results don't change following manipulation, start the diagnosis over again. For example, in the case of quasi-calcified fibrosis of a pleurovertebral ligament following tuberculosis, very precise manipulation does permit improvement of blood flow. At the beginning of my career in Grenoble, I tested and treated many tuberculosis patients in a respiratory re-education center to confirm this fact.

THE LASÈGUE TEST

This well-known test for sciatica can be refined by my approach. Let's say that you have diagnosed a right sciatica with a positive Lasègue sign of 30°, and that other test results lead you to suspect a right renal prolapse. With one hand, flex the hip to evaluate the Lasègue sign, and with the other gently push the lower pole of the right kidney superomedially *(Illustration 1-5)*. If this pushing results in gradually increased flexion at the hip on the side of the sciatica, you have confirmed renal participation in the pathological process.

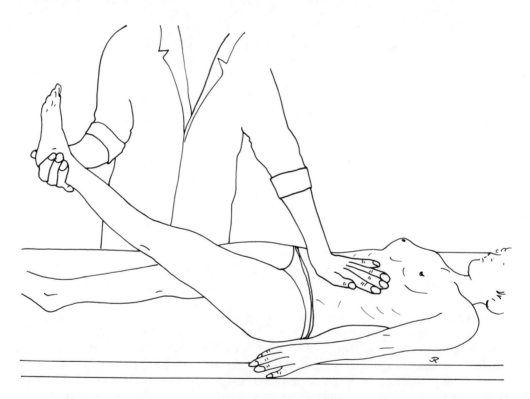

Illustration 1-5
Completed Lasègue Test

The Lasègue test can also utilize inhibition points. This approach enables one to confirm a diagnosis and avoid falling into the classic "sciatica = L4/L5 or L5/S1" trap. Experienced osteopaths know that there are numerous other possible causes and that it is better to avoid manipulation in this region in acute cases.

A genuine disc protrusion produces strong and rapid pain within the first 30° of hip flexion and is not modified by inhibition points. The Lasègue technique can be performed on all organs and articulations and is a valuable addition to our diagnostic testing arsenal. For example, you may suspect T9 as the cause of a restriction. Use a bilateral facet inhibition point and note any Lasègue improvements. Do not allow your patient to become aware of the results that you expect to obtain; this will encourage the placebo effect. Perform this test with gentleness and share your conclusions only when the technique is completed. Use of inhibition points will quickly let you know if your treatment has any chance of succeeding.

GLENOHUMERAL ARTICULATION TEST

The shoulder often reflects latent visceral pathologies. Glenohumeral periarthritis can be of traumatic origin following a fall on the shoulder, elbow, or hand, or arise from irritation of the cervical or brachial plexus. However, it is most frequently of reflex origin. In order to find evidence of a visceral restriction, I use the glenohumeral articulation test, which is performed with the patient seated and consists of testing the abduction and external rotation of the arm with one hand while creating a visceral inhibition point with the other.

Take the example of a right glenohumeral periarthritis in which you suspect involvement of the liver. First test the abduction and external rotation of the right arm. Next, lift the liver slightly (see chapter 5). If you obtain an increase in mobility of 20% or more, you can say that the cause of the shoulder problem is the liver, or the right kidney which is attached to it.

If your suspicions tend toward the cervical spine, test the irritated shoulder with one hand and, with the other, create an inhibition point on the intervertebral joint of the cervical vertebra which you found to be restricted during mobility testing. An improvement of mobility verifies that the cause is the cervical restriction (which could in turn be only a reflex). You will be surprised by the resulting improvements in mobility in such cases. Usually transient, they are merely indications for further treatment.

RADIOGRAPHY

Radiography is indispensable for diagnosis of physiological organ diseases, and can also provide important information concerning mechanical visceral problems. I shall discuss here the interpretation of X-rays of both gastric and renal prolapse.

As you can see, prolapse is well displayed by X-rays. But interpretation must include attention to important nuances. For example, Illustrations 1-6 and 1-7 show a 35-year-old man who was longilineal and suffered from dyspepsia. In the upright position (Illustration 1-6), the gastric prolapse has a sock form, with its lesser tuberosity in the pelvic area. The X-ray in the supine position (Illustration 1-7) shows that the stomach quickly finds its original form, and thus that it is not fixed on the neighboring organs. If in the supine position the lower part of the lesser tuberosity remains pelvic, it signifies a bigger problem, i.e., the stomach must be fixed to neighboring structures such as the greater omentum, small intestine, peritoneum, or bladder. The fixed stomach is often the origin of more serious gastric problems. My conclusions in looking at these X-rays are quite different from those of the gastrointestinal specialists who are only vaguely interested in this type of problem. In their minds, prolapse is not a pathological phenomenon.

Osteopaths are interested in how the viscera work as structural elements of the body; however, we should be more interested in discovering a restriction than a prolapse.

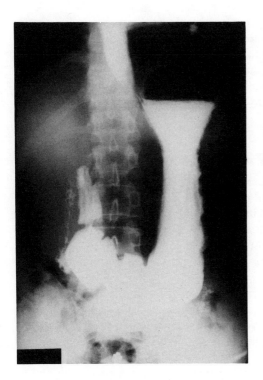 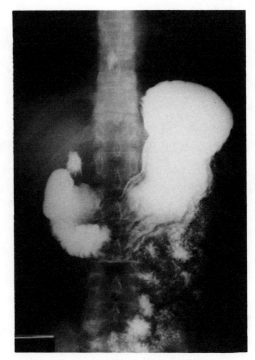

Illustration 1-6
Gastric Prolapse (Standing Position)

Illustration 1-7
Gastric Prolapse (Supine Position)

A prolapse by itself is of no great importance, but when accompanied by a fixation it becomes pathological. The osteopathic concept gives little importance to position. One only looks for mobility. I do not put the emphasis on lifting an organ, but on restoring its mobility; of course, my techniques often do have a positional effect on a visceral prolapse. For example, there are many well-documented cases of a lesser tuberosity that was originally at the level of the pubic symphysis being raised by 10cm after two or three sessions over a period of several months.

The standing kidney X-ray *(Illustration 1-8)*, from a scoliotic young nulliparous woman, shows a renal prolapse without obvious cause. The patient had urinary problems with recurrent urinary tract infections. The X-ray taken in the supine position showed the kidney remaining in exactly the same position, proving that it was fixed. A very mobile, or floating, kidney poses less problems than a fixed kidney and is easier to mobilize and release. However, once a fixed kidney is mobilized, the effect is easier to maintain.

RECOIL

Recoil consists of mobilizing an organ in such a way as to either compress it or stretch its attachments as much as possible, and then suddenly letting go. This technique can be used in either diagnosis or treatment. Let us first consider the diagnostic aspect, for which this technique is sometimes used in conventional medicine. In cases of acute

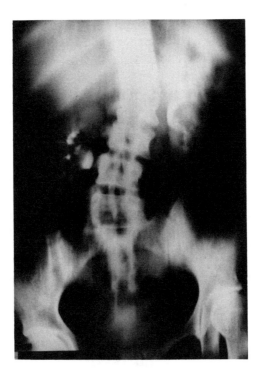

Illustration 1-8
Right Renal Prolapse

appendicitis, recoil is utilized to check for rebound tenderness, to help determine whether or not the peritoneum is affected.

As another example, consider a case in which you hesitate between diagnosing a pathology of the liver itself or of its attachments. When compression and mobilization of the organ is painful, it signifies that the organ itself is affected (e.g., viral hepatitis). If compression and mobilization cause no pain, but the sudden return to its original position does, you should think more of a ligamentous problem. Recoil is painful, e.g., with fibrosis of the suspensory ligaments of the liver.

Similarly, diaphragmatic movement can be used to expose a restriction. Pain provoked by forced inhalation (which compresses an organ in the abdominal cavity, the equivalent of direct pressure) indicates an injury to the organ. Pain provoked by forced exhalation indicates greater probability of an injury to the supporting tissues. For example, the attachments of a prolapsed kidney are stretched during exhalation and short-ened during inhalation. If the patient holds his breath for a short time during inhalation or exhalation, you can better localize the injury.

Another technique involves general stretching in backward bending. The patient is seated with both hands behind the neck, elbows close together. Standing behind him, bring the patient into a backward bending position by lifting both elbows, and maintain this position for several seconds. This stretching often reveals zones of fixation of the viscera and their attachments. The patient may be surprised by the localized areas of discomfort he feels in the trunk. Those who have tried reverse Trendelenburg tables have perhaps felt the same type of sensation. You should be able to locate irritable zones with great precision on ulcer patients. Using this technique all restrictions related to scars will reveal themselves and their different depths.

OUR RESPONSIBILITY IN DIAGNOSIS

The patients we see in osteopathic practice have not always been through other medical "filters," and we therefore have an important responsibility in terms of diagnosis. Patients suffering from joint pain may or may not have benign visceral problems, and we must be sure to distinguish which is the case. Knee and thigh pain almost always have some visceral involvement; our credibility as healers cannot remain intact with the facile generalization that all knee and back pain is due to restrictions of L3. In each of the following chapters I will describe the pathology and symptomatology of a few diseases of the organ under discussion. I have chosen those that are most common and share signs and symptoms with the functional problems I often treat. For example, significant thirst on awakening is frequently due to a renal problem, such as a prolapse, but can also occur in more serious pathologies. We should not become paralyzed by this responsibility in diagnosis but should, on the contrary, be encouraged to work even harder to enhance our understanding of medicine.

Treatment

Direct, indirect, and induction techniques were described in *Visceral Manipulation*. I would now like to discuss some additional techniques, modifications, and therapeutic considerations.

RECOIL

Recoil, whose diagnostic value was discussed above, can also provide a means of treating a restriction. The technique consists of bringing a tissue to the apex of its course and then suddenly releasing it. I think that the effect occurs through nerve reflex. The stretching and abrupt release of a structure causes the muscular and membranous tensions surrounding it to relax. This is easy to understand when a muscle is involved, but more difficult in the case of fascia. Recoil is very effective in relaxing the spasm of an organ such as the small intestine. The muscles of the intestine react well to mechanical provocations (Bayliss' law). Any stretching stimulates the proprioceptors, mechanoreceptors, and baroreceptors, which have well-documented effects on the smooth muscle. The kidney, on the other hand, has few attachments, and these are not even contractile. How can recoil produce an effect on this organ? I have not been able to discover the mechanism, but think that it may involve a reflex reaction of the posterior parietal peritoneum and Toldt's fascia.

I regard the recoil technique by itself as having only a transient effect. My colleagues Chauffour, Guillot and Guionnet use it as their principal treatment modality, and one must admit that their results are excellent, but nobody else using the same approach has achieved comparable results. Recoil, by producing immediate relaxation, increases our ability to reach and manipulate the desired organ or tissues. Stimulation of the proprioceptors facilitates topographical awareness of the body, and the body focuses its response toward the area of the restriction. I use recoil at the beginning of treatment and often at the end, to focus the body's awareness of the main viscera treated.

GENERAL INDUCTION

This technique, the therapeutic counterpart of general listening, consists of letting the body "express itself" in such a way that resolution of a restriction or series of restrictions occurs. John Upledger, D.O., taught me about unwinding, which utilizes the craniosacral system. "General induction" refers to the same approach applied to the visceral system.

While the supine position can be used, I have found the seated position to be much more effective in visceral general induction. The patient sits with the legs hanging down and the hands resting on the thighs. Stand behind him, placing your right and left hands under the liver and stomach respectively. It is important that the patient remain essentially passive, maintaining just enough muscle tone to remain precariously balanced in an upright position. In other words, the patient should relax but not collapse.

At first you should also be passive, allowing your hands to follow the tissues, exactly as in general listening. Gradually and subtly encourage the motions that you feel, increasing them. For example, if the body rotates and sidebends slightly to the right, you should encourage this motion so that it is increased. Your hands are used at the beginning to reveal the unconscious motions of the body, and later to amplify these motions.

The patient will turn around your fingers, which are used to detect and release the restrictions; i.e., your fingers not only find the restrictions about which the body is turning, but also act to mobilize those areas locally through direct stretching in the opposite direction. In a synergistic fashion, you should use the spontaneous motion of the body in concert with the stretching effects of your fingers on the restriction. This in turn helps resolve the spontaneous motion of the body. For example, if there is a restriction between the transverse colon and the liver near the right triangular ligament, the body may rotate to the left while your fingers are stretching the affected area to the right. As the technique progresses you will feel a melding between your hands and the patient's body so that they feel like a single entity.

The motion will initially become more and more rapid, increase in amplitude, or both. It will then gradually slow down and/or decrease in amplitude as the restrictions are released. Finally the motion stops, almost as if you had released an accumulation of energy in the body. After this the general visceral motion will have good amplitude, vitality and symmetry. The body will be peaceful and the patient should remain quiet for a few minutes.

It is important to know when the technique is finished. Do not stop until the spontaneous motion of the body stops by itself and there is also a local release of the tissues involved. This technique allows the body to speak directly, but if the technique is overly prolonged, or the motion becomes too rapid or the amplitude too great, the movements cease being passive expressions of the patient's inherent physical restrictions and become active movements ordered by the patient's mind. If this happens, very strong psychological reactions may occur. For example, about ten years ago I needed the help of two colleagues to restrain a patient who became so violent after treatment that he tried to break all the furniture in the office. It took us over 30 minutes to calm him down. Such incidents are rare, but do occur. While I recognize that the barrier between mind and body is very fragile, I generally prefer to stay at the physical level. I avoid provoking strong psychological reactions, as I do not have the necessary training to treat psychiatric problems. My only aim is to release visceral restrictions.

In American osteopathy a similar type of general induction, applied to the craniosacral system, is called "unwinding." This is an appropriate term in that the process is similar to the unwinding of a bobbin or tangled telephone cord, during which the primary restriction is revealed.

TREATMENT STRATEGY

In osteopathy, it is sometimes difficult to find the restriction that is the key to the patient's problem. Should one first manipulate the skull, vertebral column, viscera, or limbs? Personally, I do not believe in the inevitable discovery of the primary restriction. There are so many possible causes that we can only hope to discover the "least secondary" of these, even if we refer to it as the "primary" restriction. Nonetheless, the order of treatment is important, and I would make the following suggestions:

Do not begin treatment by an adjustment of the vertebral column, but rather by cranial and visceral techniques. Vertebral manipulation should be performed only after you have tried to free all the other zones, better enabling yourself to find the primary vertebral restriction.

Always look for restrictions of the feet and the sacrococcygeal articulation. These are particularly pathogenic for the visceral system. The importance of the sacrococcygeal joint was discussed in chapter 11 of *Visceral Manipulation*. I often find foot restrictions in patients with visceral problems. I can think of two reasons for this. One is the neurological connection: many abdominal and pelvic organs are innervated by nerves that also go to the lower extremities, and disorders in one area can therefore have a reflex effect on the other. There are also mechanical connections: visceral restrictions upset the balance of soft tissues which affect the stance and, therefore, the feet. Conversely, problems of the feet may have a cascade effect that upsets the mechanics of the viscera.

When there are several restrictions (particularly in the upper abdomen) or a large restriction (e.g., in the aftermath of peritonitis), general induction is usually preferable. For single restrictions it is better to work locally. For example, if there is only a restriction of the sphincter of Oddi, you will obtain the best results by working on that area; however, if in addition the gallbladder and right triangular ligament are involved, you should use general induction and move your fingers slightly to work on all the affected areas.

With osteopathy, one begins with local treatment and ends with general manipulation in order to harmonize the reaction of the body. When you start locally, you can be relatively discrete and gentle (thus stimulating the patient's energy), and gradually involve more and more of the body. If a practitioner (particularly a beginner) starts right in with general manipulation, there is a tendency to work too suddenly and quickly; such treatment will exhaust part of the patient's energy without stimulating the self-healing mechanisms. In other words, if you start on a general or systemic level and make a mistake, you will dissipate the energy of the patient without obtaining results and therefore waste that treatment session. However, if you start locally you can gently correct any reaction of the body which you feel is unhealthy while the patient still retains enough energy to allow continuation of the treatment.

The general state of the patient's energy is a very important determinant of the success of the treatment. Of all the visceral manipulative techniques, motility is the one that interacts most with the patient's energy. For this reason I end treatment sessions by working on motility. Of course, this does not imply that motility is more important than mobility, nor does it allow you to skip treatments for mobility. Without the ability to move freely and smoothly through its anatomical environment, an organ cannot attain good motility.

Osteopathic treatment should not be overly prolonged. Never ask a patient to come on a weekly basis over a period of many months. This is particularly true when working on the deep energy of the body through such organs as the liver and kidneys. If you work on these often (even on a weekly basis) instead of letting the body do the work, you may get good results initially, but the body will soon stop responding. The excretory canals, such as the gallbladder, sphincter of Oddi and cecum, can be worked on every week without ill effect; however, I still believe that such frequent treatment is unnecessary.

Osteopathy is not a form of "nursing," wherein you work without letting the patient's body express itself. Your hands must stimulate and inform the body, without ever replacing it. The often-quoted statement by A.T. Still, "find it, fix it and leave it alone," means for our purposes that you must find the restriction, treat it, and then let the body carry on from there. M. Michallet's experiments, described below, demonstrate that the effects of manipulation continue over time.

TREATMENT OF CHILDREN

Infants and small children require special consideration and gentleness. They are especially cherished patients, not only because of their delicacy, but also because we can learn so much from them. For example, I have observed that at the exact moment that the umbilical cord is cut in newborns and they become dependent on the external environment for oxygen, there is a strong restriction of T4 as the lungs come into action. This has deepened my appreciation of the mechanics of breathing. It is interesting to listen to the motility of the mother's uterus post partum and compare it to the general motion of the baby's tissues—you can usually deduce the position of the baby *in utero*. This underscores the fact that the tissues have an active memory.

In general, I do not treat mobility in infants as there is a real risk of damaging the organs, especially the liver, which is relatively large and delicate. I have to admit that I myself have made this mistake. When a child is over seven months old and has begun to roll around and/or crawl, you can begin to work with mobility as long as you do so with extreme gentleness. Even when using induction, be very careful, since applying too much pressure can create restrictions that are difficult to resolve.

I often use visceral manipulation in the treatment of children. The liver and kidneys are very important organs in children. I treat the liver in cases of recurrent infections, chronic fever, poor digestion, hypotonia, and dehydration. Children who are weak or whose development is delayed usually benefit from kidney manipulation, as do those with problems of the lower limbs. I combine treatment of the kidneys and bladder for enuresis.

In my experience the most common restrictions in young children affect the cranium, shoulders and digestive system. For the first of these, cranial treatment is most effective; induction is recommended for the other two. I prefer to work on small children with the feet in my right hand and the head in my left. For example, to treat the very common right first rib problem I twist the legs and lower body to the left to focus on the rib.

In children there is a strong link between problems of the digestive organs and cranial restrictions. Often, after two or three visceral manipulation sessions, I have observed the disappearance of reflux, regurgitation, and other malfunctions in infants. These could be resolved as well by cranial manipulation. I usually treat such cases with one hand over the stomach (specifically the hiatus) and the other over the lower occiput (foramen magnum). The technique consists of establishing a smooth connection between the two hands. At the beginning of a treatment session when you pull the dura cephalad (using a slight "induction-like" pressure), the hiatus moves posteriorly; by the end of the session this does not occur.

Honesty obliges me to point out the frequent occurrence of neurological immaturity of various sphincters, which often resolves as time goes by. However, I have obtained results immediately after treatment sessions, which to me indicates a cause and effect relationship.

I have had much success treating relatively mild cases of pyloric stenosis; however, if the child cannot swallow without vomiting, manipulation is not useful. During treatment, it is important to have one hand anterior and the other posterior, working through both hands in both the transverse and sagittal planes.

Children with tenderness of the hepatic and splenic flexures or the sigmoid colon often have parasites. These are more common in the industrialized countries than most people think. Parasite-infested children will usually pick their nose, scratch various parts of their body (often including the anus, forearms, or eyelids), pull their ears, etc.

For children with chronic sinusitis (a common disorder), I order removal of all dairy products from the diet. Treatment aimed at improving the motility of the liver is often successful. On the other hand, I believe that children with chronic sore throats have problems of the immune system, and have used induction of the thymus and appendix very successfully in these cases.

Low back pain in children is rarely due to musculoskeletal causes. In children with low back pain, check the function of the viscera of the lower abdomen carefully; you will almost always find the cause there.

Babies always cry for a reason. A child who cries repeatedly should be checked thoroughly.

JACQUES-MARIE MICHALLET'S RESEARCH

One problem in osteopathy is that we observe clinical results but are usually unable to document them in an objective fashion. The kidneys, however, are easily detected by ultrasonography, and their mobility can thus be precisely measured. Jacques-Marie Michallet used ultrasound to study the effects of visceral manipulation on the kidneys as his thesis project for his Diploma of Osteopathy here in France. I was honored to serve as his sponsor, and we are grateful to the imaging specialist Dr. Serge Cohen of Grenoble for making this research possible (see Appendix).

Michallet selected 25 subjects (seven men and 18 women) who had been treated by various osteopaths for presumed renal ptoses with symptoms such as extreme fatigue, dizzy spells, back pain, abdominal distention, muscular spasms, problems with arterial pressure, etc. The proportion of men and women in this study was fairly typical of that in our practice. Generally 60% of our cases are women, but with renal cases the proportion is closer to 70% (see chapter 9).

Because air in the colic flexures interferes with ultrasound, mobility of the right kidney was measured at its superior pole and that of the left kidney at its inferior pole. Mobility was measured after several forced inhalations and exhalations and the largest measurement was recorded. Of the 25 cases, 24 involved the right kidney; prolapse of the left kidney is quite rare.

Michallet's goal was to gather objective data concerning the extent of kidney mobility following manipulation. Some of the patients had previous intravenous urography showing strong evidence of a positive renal prolapse that subsequent ultrasonography failed to reveal. With the patient in a seated position, the kidneys were manipulated at about 7 P.M., before dinner. This time was chosen because the effects of gravity during the day increase ptosis (accentuating the problem), and because the abdomen is most easily manipulated when the stomach is empty.

In every case, the mobility of the treated kidney showed an immediate increase in amplitude (mean 17.2 mm). The increase was less striking in brevilineal patients. Michallet did not stop at this stage of experimentation, but asked the patients to come back two months later. Of the 25 patients, 18 complied; in 16 of them Michallet observed a further, delayed increase in mobility (mean 8.6 mm). Thus, the mean increase in mobility among these 16 patients was 25.8 mm!

The protocol for this experiment was quite strict. Dr. Cohen imposed many precautions to avoid any artifacts or placebo effects. Under these circumstances, the probability that the observed increase in mobility was due to chance is very low. These results bear witness to the undeniable effects of manipulation on the mobility of an organ. Some therapists had assured me that it was impossible to reach a kidney manually by the anterior route! I had to demonstrate the technique numerous times with fluoroscopy in order for them to ultimately accept the facts.

The delayed effect which was noted is proof that one needs merely to give the information to the body and to free the restriction, not treat the patient repeatedly over a prolonged period. We have nothing to do with re-education; let the body correct itself. From my experience, treatment once every three weeks seems to be enough, and positive results should be observable within four sessions. If not, the osteopathic treatment should be modified, or totally abandoned in favor of other approaches.

Plexuses of the Autonomic Nervous System

These have an important role in visceral manipulation, but do not fit comfortably elsewhere in this book. I will therefore discuss them here.

When performing visceral manipulation I often begin my work by focusing working on adhesions, fixations, fibrosis, etc.; that is, I start by working on the mobility of a specific organ. When the mobility has been normalized, I then work on the motility of that organ. In other words, I work discretely and get a discrete response from the body. In order to spread the effect through the body, it is necessary to stimulate and utilize the nervous system, which is the primary integrative system of the body. This is an important step: mobilizing the liver does not have much effect if the response does not involve the entire body.

For this purpose I use the larger plexuses of the autonomic nervous system, which are aggregations of nerves and ganglia in the trunk. It is not uncommon to find a small amount of adrenal tissue in the plexuses, which reflects their embryological development. Nerves from these plexuses innervate the viscera. The three largest plexuses are the cardiac, celiac (also known as solar) and inferior hypogastric, each of which gives rise to numerous minor plexuses for the specific organs and structures innervated.

ANATOMY

Because the celiac plexus is the largest of the major autonomic plexuses, I will describe it in some detail. It is made up of two celiac ganglia located posteriorly to the stomach, the spigelian lobe of the liver and the omental bursa. They are anterior to the crura of the diaphragm, the beginning of the abdominal aorta, and the inferior vena cava (this is at the level of T10-12 and L1). The ganglia are bordered medially by the celiac trunk, and the net of nerves which issues from them surrounds the celiac trunk and its branches.

The celiac ganglia are irregularly shaped and grayish red in color. The superior part of each ganglion is joined by the greater splanchnic nerve while the inferior part receives the lesser splanchnic nerve. The two celiac ganglia are connected by the greater and lesser splanchnic nerves of both sides, as well as some fibers from the vagus and phrenic nerves. From a clinical point of view, they therefore form a single plexus. Efferent branches go in front of the aorta and all around the celiac trunk and the superior mesenteric artery. The celiac plexus sends rami to almost all the abdominal organs and the abdominal wall. These rami follow and surround the different arteries and form secondary plexuses, such as the phrenic, hepatic, left gastric, splenic, adrenal, renal, abdominal aortic, inferior mesenteric, and ovarian.

The celiac plexus is sometimes called the "abdominal brain" because it regulates all the abdominal organs. An injury to the plexus can provoke syncope and, very rarely, death. Irritation of the plexus after peritonitis or mechanical inflammation can lead to cardiac, respiratory, intestinal, renal or adrenal problems.

The surface projection for listening to the celiac plexus is located just to the right of the intersection between the midline and the transverse line connecting the ninth costochondral joints (usually 2cm below the xiphoid process). Anatomically speaking, one would not expect this to be so, inasmuch as the celiac plexus is composed of small ganglia that are spread over a larger area than this point. However, in terms of local listening, the best information about the plexus is obtained from this rather specific location. The celiac plexus can also be located by using manual pressure, since compression always results in epigastric pain.

The hypogastric plexus is made up of two bilateral ganglia located at the inferior part of the posterior bladder, cervix and uterosacral ligaments in women, and at the inferior part of the posterior bladder and lateral rectum in men. The plexuses are formed by the hypogastric nerve and branches from the pelvic splanchnic nerves. The hypogastric plexus sends fibers to the pelvic viscera, either directly or by accompanying the branches of the internal iliac artery. Even though some of these fibers innervate the descending and sigmoid colon, this plexus is also known as the "urogenital brain." To work on the inferior hypogastric plexus, place the hand on the pubic symphysis so that your palm is directly anterior to the sacrum.

The cardiac plexus is divided into two parts. The superficial part, located just below the aortic arch and anterior to the right pulmonary artery, is formed by branches from the superior cervical ganglion and from the left vagus. The deep part of the cardiac plexus is anterior to the tracheal bifurcation and posterior to the aortic arch. It is formed by branches from the cervical and upper thoracic ganglia of the sympathetic trunk, and branches from the vagus and recurrent laryngeal nerves. The cardiac plexus primarily sends fibers to the different parts of the heart and the coronary arteries, as well as to the great vessels of the thorax. The anterior surface projection of the cardiac plexus is at the level of the first and second left sternocostal joints. On listening, put your palm on the fifth left costochondral joints and your fingers on the first and second joints, so that the hand is obliquely directed up and to the right. If you place your hand sagittally you will be picking up information from the joints, not the plexus.

PATHOLOGY

When a plexus is in a state of hyperactivity, it will discharge its excess energy in order to regain balance. Depending on the patient, this discharge can go to the musculoskeletal, craniosacral, or visceral systems. If a structure is weak, it will tend to be overstimulated and adversely affected by this discharge. For example, in cases of gastritis with a hyperactive celiac plexus, the stomach will receive the largest part of the discharge from the plexus, which will exacerbate the gastritis, leading to further stimulation of the celiac plexus, and so on in a vicious circle.

The celiac plexus is integrally related to the emotions. Very often the first emotional response of the body goes through the celiac plexus to the gallbladder or stomach. For example, when you hear bad news such as "your car was stolen," your gallbladder immediately spasms and you feel a contraction in the upper part of the abdomen. This spasm does not usually present a danger to the body; on the contrary, it gives the mind a pathway to eliminate some of the emotional tension. However, if the process is sustained or chronic it will adversely affect the body.

OSTEOPATHIC DIAGNOSIS

When the celiac plexus attracts the hand on local listening, the heel of the hand ends about 2cm below and slightly to the right of the xiphoid process, with the fingers on the sternum. Usually with local listening you know that you are on the site of the restriction when your hand reaches a place where it becomes immobile. However, when you reach any of the autonomic nervous plexuses your hand will rock, either from side to side, or back to front. In mild cases the motion is approximately 15 cycles per minute and is, of course, unrelated to the breathing cycle. The greater the amplitude and frequency of the motion, the higher the state of nervous tension in the patient. If a plexus is functioning normally, it will not attract the hand at all on local listening.

To focus your local listening on a plexus, first place your hand over the surface projection of that plexus and press slightly posteriorly. Then release the pressure so that the only force applied is the weight of your hand. When you become attuned to the motion of the plexus you will feel a superficial, wave-like motion on the skin as described above. Listening to an organ is different from listening to a plexus. When listening to an organ you are visualizing its anatomy and focusing on its physiology as precisely as possible. When listening to a plexus you are trying to hold in your mind a picture of the patient's entire organism. Looking at the patient's face will sometimes increase your awareness of psychological factors and make this task easier.

Often our diagnostic techniques lead us to an autonomic nervous plexus. The basis for this attraction is unclear, as is the mechanism for the rocking motion. These surface projections of the plexuses are certainly "energy" areas; however, the nature of the energy is not clear.

TREATMENT

The autonomic plexuses are treated by a form of induction. First you tune into the rocking motion and go with it, as in induction of an organ. As you do this, the frequency and amplitude of the motion will increase for awhile. Then, without any active intervention on your part, the amplitude will decrease and the frequency will diminish until it either slows down to less than 15 cycles per minute, or stops altogether. The release that follows induction of a plexus can be sudden and dramatic. For this treatment technique to work, you must have a light touch and be able to follow the motion closely.

I usually work first on the celiac plexus. After the release I then do local listening at a very superficial level to see if my hand is attracted superiorly or inferiorly. If it is attracted superiorly, I work on the cardiac plexus; if inferiorly, I work on the inferior hypogastric plexus. Induction of the plexuses can be performed at the very beginning of a treatment session if the patient is so anxious that his body does not respond to other techniques. This treatment is useful in preparing the patient for other techniques because it relieves spasms of both the visceral system (gallbladder, pylorus, sphincter of Oddi, etc.) and musculoskeletal system. I have found that it also facilitates obtaining a good response to craniosacral techniques. In general, however, induction of the plexuses is performed at the end of a treatment session in order to balance the body's energy.

At the end of a visceral treatment, especially one in which you have concentrated too narrowly on a specific component of the body, there may be too much activity or energy in a small area. Balancing both the abdominal plexuses helps to harmonize and balance the body's energy, allowing the body to respond generally to the treatment and to integrate this response at the psychological and emotional levels. Put one hand on the celiac plexus and the other on the hypogastric plexus. Let each hand follow the rocking motion of its plexus. Allow the amplitude and frequency of the motion to increase; then follow it as it slows down until both hands have stopped. *(Illustration 1-9)*. This is also an excellent means of relaxing a patient, either before or after other treatment. Because this technique may have strong psychological and emotional effects, it can lead to fairly intense emotional releases, so be prepared.

Recommendations

Each chapter in this book will conclude with recommendations concerning contraindications, advice to the patient, etc.

The absolute contraindications involve those organic lesions for which manipulation presents the risk of initiating an invasive process or causing vascular injury. For example, manipulation of a duodenal ulcer which is beginning to perforate could cause hemorrhage. Chapter 4 presents a detailed discussion of clinical symptoms of the stomach and duodenum which demand caution.

Another contraindication of abdominal manipulation is an aneurysm of the abdominal aorta. I have encountered several cases of aortic aneurysm in my practice and believe that this discovery and the subsequent surgery saved the life of the patients. You should be able to recognize aneurysms so that direct manipulation, which could be dangerous for the patient, can be avoided. I have never heard of manipulation leading to rupture of an aneurysm, but the walls of some aneurysms are so thin that this risk must be considered.

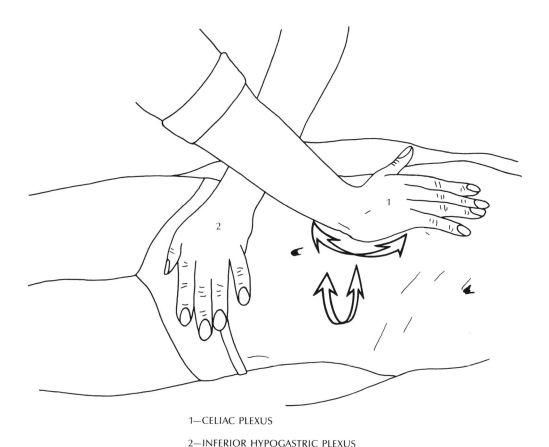

1—CELIAC PLEXUS

2—INFERIOR HYPOGASTRIC PLEXUS

Illustration 1-9
Listening: Autonomic Plexuses

Most aneurysms occur between the point where the renal arteries branch off and the bifurcation of the abdominal aorta into the two common iliac arteries *(Illustration 1-10)*. They are rare but very dangerous. It has been estimated that the risk of death when the diameter of the aneurysm is 6 cm is roughly 25% during the first year and 50% within five years, or 50% and 90% respectively when the diameter is much greater than 6 cm. Most aneurysm patients have no consistent symptoms, although if the aneurysm happens to occur near the inferior duodenum the patient may experience upper abdominal pain, nausea and vomiting.

On abdominal palpation of a patient with an aneurysm, you will feel distinct abdominal pulsations and a pulsatile mass that crosses the midline. The mass is painless but the pulsations will often be uncomfortable when the patient lies in the prone position. Sometimes there are also signs of arterial insufficiency in the lower limbs. Occasionally there will be back pain due to compression of the spinal cord or spinal nerves. An expansion of the aneurysm can manifest as acute lumbar pain. In conclusion, be very cautious if you feel a large, pulsatile mass that crosses the midline, particularly if the patient is having low back pain that is not affected by movement. In such cases an aneurysm must be suspected and ultrasound is strongly indicated.

Another important point is that while patients may experience some tenderness during visceral manipulation, there should never be severe pain. If there is, stop the manipulation immediately and determine the reason for the pain. If you cannot do so, refer the patient to someone who can.

Advice to patients should reflect your clinical experience and lead to prevention of avoidable recurrences. Improving the subclavian circulation of a patient who, later that day, paints a ceiling, will not be particularly helpful. The patient must be careful in how he uses his body. Nonetheless, apart from a few specific movements to be avoided, I usually recommend to my patients that they change nothing in their normal physical routine.

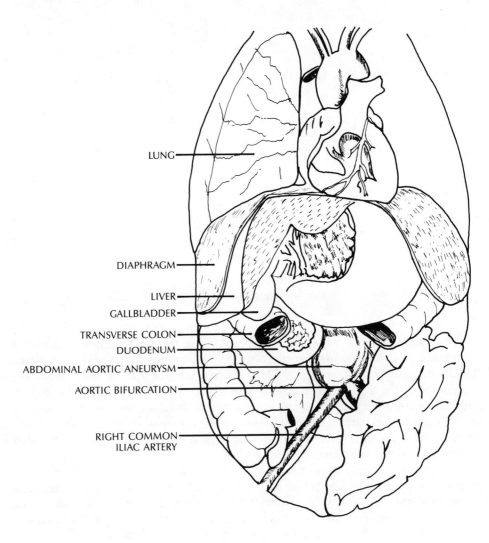

LUNG

DIAPHRAGM

LIVER

GALLBLADDER

TRANSVERSE COLON

DUODENUM

ABDOMINAL AORTIC ANEURYSM

AORTIC BIFURCATION

RIGHT COMMON
ILIAC ARTERY

Illustration 1-10
Aneurysm of the Abdominal Aorta

Some patients with low back pain whose cause is neither discovered nor treated may be obliged to live at a slower pace for several years in order to prevent a recurrence. Osteopathic treatments, which address the cause, can make this change in lifestyle unnecessary. Be careful with your advice and always assume that it will be followed; it should not be harmful to the physical harmony of the patient, nor pointlessly restrictive.

I believe that all problems come about from the compensation of the body to chronic stresses. Treatment should be aimed at relieving those stresses and less concerned with the effects of recent trauma. For example, I live in an area surrounded by the Alps, yet I see more instances of acute low back pain resulting from bending to pick up small objects than from skiing dangerously.

Chapter Two:
The Peritoneum

Table of Contents

The Peritoneum

Problems with peritoneal structures rarely constitute a primary or causal pathology; however, these structures are almost always affected by problems of the abdominal organs, including laparotomy, infection and trauma. In this chapter I shall augment the anatomical descriptions in *Visceral Manipulation* and describe several mobilization techniques for the peritoneum. These techniques should be performed after treatment of other organs because the latter act via the peritoneum and often cause restrictions there. The greater omentum and anterior parietal peritoneum are manipulated by the same techniques.

Greater Omentum

This division of the peritoneum originates as two visceral peritoneal folds covering the anterior and posterior surfaces of the stomach; the two folds unite at the greater curvature of the stomach and descend from there. The greater omentum then spreads out to cover most of the anterior surface of the small intestine, folds back on itself, and runs upward to attach to the anterior surface of the transverse colon *(Illustration 2-1)*. It is continuous with the visceral peritoneum of the transverse colon and thereby with the mesocolon, which attaches the colon to the posterior parietal peritoneum at the level of the kidneys. Laterally, the attachments of the greater omentum are often confused with the phrenicocolic ligaments.

The greater omentum is riddled with numerous vascular orifices, carries the vessels which supply the stomach, and is normally laden with adipose tissue which makes it easy to find upon dissection. It can be described as having four edges and two surfaces. The upper edge is fixed to the transverse colon, to the greater curvature of the stomach, and often to the phrenicocolic ligaments. The lateral edges rest upon the ascending and descending colons. The irregular lower edge hangs above the pubis and inguinal ligament, extending farther down on the left. The anterior and posterior surfaces face the anterior abdominal wall and the small intestine respectively.

The greater omentum undeniably has a mechanical protective role in the abdomen, i.e., acts as a shock absorber. It also has an important vascular function in the digestive system, as evidenced by the numerous vessels running through and across it. The adipose layer acts as an insulator, preventing rapid gain or loss of heat from the intestines. The

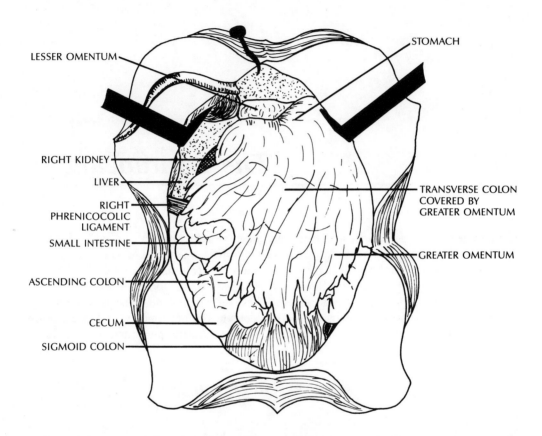

Illustration 2-1
Greater Omentum

greater omentum also contains large numbers of lymph nodes and therefore has an immune function; it is affected by conditions such as appendicitis, other abdominal infections, tuberculosis, and abdominal cancers.

MECHANICAL PROBLEMS

The greater omentum falls easily into the hernial "tracts" and often constitutes the major portion of hernias associated with the small intestine. As it extends lower down on the left, it penetrates more easily into the left hernial tracts.

Since it is often involved in cases of infection, the greater omentum can also create adhesions. Those affecting the small intestine can disturb intestinal transit, and produce a harmful effect on abdominal vascular circulation, particularly during periods of digestion or intense physical activity. These adhesions can also disturb intestinal mobility and motility. When you walk, bend over, etc., the intestine must be able to move freely within the abdominal cavity. A restriction of the greater omentum prevents this movement from taking place and produces spasms of the digestive and circulatory systems. When a patient has acute pain after running, consider a mechanical problem of the greater omentum. If pain diminishes during digestion or after physical effort, think more of a reflex vascular abdominal problem originating in the greater omentum.

For various reasons, such as a prolapse of the stomach or transverse colon, the greater omentum can also prolapse. With a freely mobile prolapse, the patient feels only slight abdominal discomfort. However, if it is fixed by adhesions, the effects are more disabling, and may affect the digestive or urinary organs.

Prolapses of the greater omentum and stomach typically occur together and produce the same clinical symptoms. There is pulling of the phrenicocolic ligaments, which causes spasms of the colic flexures and accumulation of air in the colon. Movement of the diaphragm is affected, particularly with exhalation, because it is during this phase that there is an increase in tension of these structures.

Parietal Peritoneum

The peritoneum is by far the most complex of the serous membranes. Its visceral portion covers the abdominal organs and forms structures such as the greater omentum and mesentery, while its parietal portion lines the abdominal cavity. Visceral manipulation requires the ability to reach and treat the parietal peritoneum.

Anteroinferiorly, the parietal peritoneum is supported by the median and medial umbilical ligaments *(Visceral Manipulation, p. 220)*. Thin at the front, it thickens posteriorly, particularly in the lumbar area, and is lined by a subperitoneal adipose layer.

A part of the peritoneum called mesothelium secretes serous fluid which facilitates movement of the organs and sliding of the parietal and visceral layers. If there is irritation or infection, secretion of this fluid may increase considerably and it becomes more viscous. This is why adhesions can develop very quickly, sometimes within only a few hours.

Surgical procedures often cause restrictions of the peritoneum. Laparoscopy often causes anterior peritoneal adhesions, usually 3-4 cm below the umbilicus. These adhesions can lead to many problems, which are manifested when the patient bends backward. Because this moves the umbilicus farther from the pubis and stretches the anterior peritoneum, it will provoke pain at the point of restriction.

These adhesions are often the cause of visceral mechanical disturbances, as they disrupt sliding between the organs. Stretching of organs and ligaments then causes local pain and vascular spasms which disturb the patient and lead him to seek treatment. Because there are no objective signs, the symptom is treated as subjective and the patient as a hypochondriac. One such patient who complained of acute abdominal pain during digestion was found, on post-mortem dissection (which I participated in), to have numerous abdominal adhesions which could have disturbed vascular circulation and intestinal transit.

Diagnosis of Restrictions

It is not possible to distinguish with the fingers between the greater omentum and anterior parietal peritoneum, both of which are located just deep to the abdominal muscles. They are spread out like a cloth and to test them you must choose two pressure points, the first being a fixed point and the second chosen to enable you to stretch the peritoneum and evaluate its elasticity. In order to avoid muscular contractions, you must initially choose pressure points at the intersection of muscles.

Anteriorly, such points are found along the external edges of the rectus abdominis muscle, directly underneath the costal attachments of the abdominal muscles, along the midline and inguinal ligament, and around the umbilicus. Laterally, such points are found in a triangular area bounded by the anterior edge of the latissimus dorsi, posterior edge of the external abdominal oblique muscle, and iliac crest. The posterior points are in Grynfeltt's triangle (also known as Lesshaft's space), which is bounded superiorly by R12 and the serratus posterior muscle, posteriorly by the quadratus lumborum, and anteriorly by the posterior edge of the internal abdominal oblique muscle.

LISTENING

Local listening can also be utilized here. To listen to the anterior peritoneum and greater omentum, put your two index fingers and thumbs at the superolateral and inferolateral aspects, respectively, of the rectus abdominis muscle, and focus on the anterior part of the body. For the lateral aspect of the peritoneum, the thumbs and index fingers are similarly placed but the little fingers are located as far laterally as possible. To listen to the posterior peritoneum, the middle fingers are placed just lateral to the transverse process of L3, and the rest of the hands on the posterolateral aspects of the trunk. If your hands are big enough, you can listen to the entire peritoneum without moving your hands. Local listening is performed as discussed in chapter 1, i.e., your hands and mind are passive and attracting the patient's body. If there are problems with the peritoneum, they will usually be at the "corners" of the box formed by your hands (e.g., the right superolateral corner of the rectus abdominis). Always listen to the peritoneum after completing your other techniques.

DISTENSIBILITY TEST

This test involves fixing part of the peritoneum with one hand and stretching with the other, trying to eliminate all muscular participation by working between two muscles or two layers of muscles. It can be performed in either the seated (Illustration 2-2) or supine position.

For the anterosuperior test, place the fingers of your left hand on the left superolateral edge of the rectus abdominis and push them slightly posterior. The fingers of your right hand are symmetrically placed on the right superolateral edge of the same muscle. Either move one hand away from the other (which is being used as a fixed point), or move both of them away from each other, stretching the peritoneum. Try to avoid any participation of the small intestine by not pushing too far posteriorly.

For another variation of this test, leave your left fingers in the superior position as described above and place the right hand on the inferolateral edge of the rectus abdominis, near the ileocecal junction or even lower. Stretch these two zones to evaluate the distensibility of the peritoneum. Alternatively, you can exert pressure at a point below the xiphoid and at another just behind the pubic symphysis and stretch the peritoneum between these points. There are many other possible variations to this test which I shall leave to your imagination.

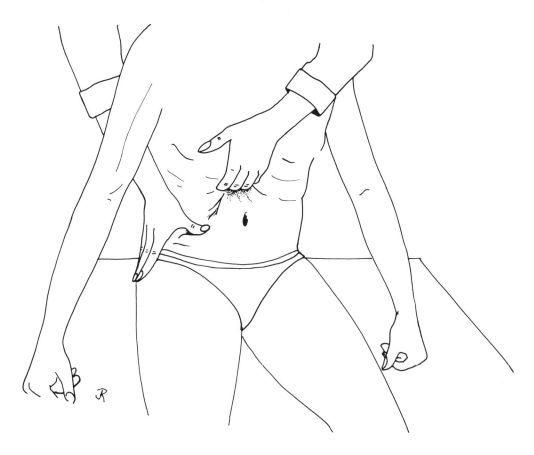

Illustration 2-2
Peritoneal Distensibility Test (Seated Position)

Two important considerations are to avoid any involvement of adjacent viscera, and to cover the largest surface possible in order to obtain a true stretching effect, as if straightening out a tablecloth. Compare the elasticity of the left plane with that of the right plane, remembering that the omentum covers more of the left part of the abdomen.

Be aware of what the patient is feeling. The parietal peritoneum receives sensory fibers from the phrenic nerve, vagus nerve and lumbar plexus; stretching should not be painful. Pain is often an indication of a restriction. Sometimes the patient is aware of deeper sensations which indicate zones of adhesion of other peritoneal folds (e.g., mesocolon, mesentery, lesser omentum). These folds are tested in the same manner as the viscera which they partition and support.

MOTILITY TEST

Peritoneal motility tests can be performed with the patient in the supine position with legs bent, or in the seated position. In the supine position *(Illustration 2-3)*, place your two hands flat, fingers spread, on either side of the midline. Only their weight should be felt; let them listen. When the peritoneum is free of any adhesion or restriction, your hands will perform a slight supination, as if the thumbs were lifting up and the pisiforms were pushing into the abdomen. In the case of an adhesion or restriction, the palm moves toward the affected area.

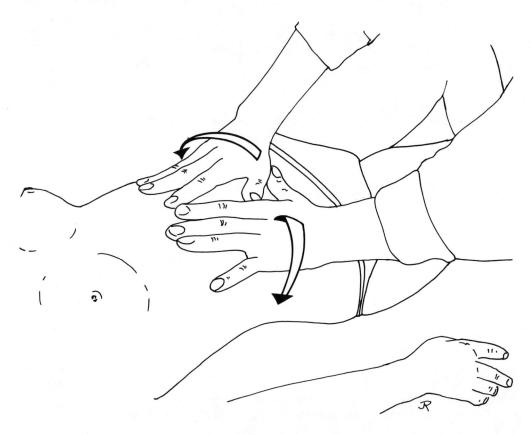

Illustration 2-3
Peritoneal Motility Test (Supine Position)

Diagnosis for lesions located more deeply involves greater pressure from the hands. If you think you have found a peritoneal restriction, increase the manual pressure. If the motility test returns to normal, the restriction is confirmed to be relatively superficial. If not, think about visceral participation, usually of the small or large intestine.

In a variation of this test, the patient is in the seated position with legs hanging down. Place your hands with the thumbs posteriorly in Grynfeltt's triangle and the fingers on the lateral part of the abdomen, avoiding the ribs. An advantage of this technique is that you have an important part of the abdomen under your fingers; however, a drawback is that it is relatively imprecise, since in this position the patient is relatively unbalanced and moves rather easily. Therefore, this version of the motility test lacks specificity. When there is restriction, you will usually feel the cylinder of the abdomen rotating around it. Corroborate this test with the supine version.

Treatment

A direct treatment technique with the patient in the supine position consists of freeing the fixed planes implicated by the diagnostic tests, using stretching with one or both hands. For example, in the case of an omental restriction around the ileocecal junction, you can fix the area under the lateral edge of the rectus abdominis facing the cecum, and use the symmetrically opposite point for stretching. You may also fix the ileocecal area and stretch the right inguinal area, following with the area found above the pubic symphysis. You may even create counter-pressure at the level of Grynfeltt's triangle, on the subcostal peritoneal attachment, in front of the left or right phrenicocolic ligament, or in any suitable area. The treatment consists of rhythmic, gentle repetition of the stretching until the tissues release. In addition to these direct manipulations, you can perform indirect ones combining rotations of the torso or the lower limbs.

As a general rule, first try to stretch the superficial planes of the abdomen. All too often, I see students direct their fingers too deeply, liberating the sagittally-oriented deep peritoneal restrictions, but neglecting the superficial restrictions. The loosening of a deep restriction may have no influence at all on a superficial restriction.

A variation of this technique is performed with the patient in the seated position, both hands joined behind the head. Let us assume again that a restriction has been localized near the ileocecal junction. You pull both elbows to bring the patient into backward bending, left sidebending and right rotation. With your free hand, fix the ileocecal zone to increase the stretching.

As noted above, the anterior and posterior portions of the greater omentum are attached to the stomach and transverse colon respectively. To mobilize the omentum, one can mobilize these two viscera. Taking a pressure point slightly medial to each colic flexure (i.e., hepatic and splenic), lift the medial parts of the flexures superolaterally. If you do not use too much pressure, you can avoid affecting the colon. At the end of the movement, bend the patient backward. The transverse colon seems little affected by this technique because of its great natural mobility.

In a third version of the direct technique, the patient rests on his knees and elbows. Stand beside and slightly behind him (right-handed people usually work better if they stand to the patient's left with this position), and place the heels of each palm just lateral to the lateral edges of the rectus abdominis, with the fingers interlaced (Illustration 2-4). Stand close to the patient so that you can use your entire body to move him instead of just the hands. Draw the palms together (sometimes pulling them posteriorly first to increase the amount of flesh you can grasp), then move them anteriorly (i.e., toward the table top) while remaining focused on the restrictions. This technique stretches the skin, peritoneum, and small intestine. Because of the great amplitude of the stretching, it affects the lateral and posterior, as well as anterior, parts of the peritoneum, and increases the efficacy of the technique. You can selectively focus on the anterior, lateral or posterior part depending upon the location and direction of the restriction. It is often helpful to perform recoil at the beginning and end of this treatment.

Although manipulation of both kidneys affects the posterior parietal peritoneum, it is difficult to obtain simultaneous mobilization. In order to free posterior peritoneal restrictions, I use stretching of the psoas muscle, diaphragm, lower ribs, or upper lumbar and lower thoracic vertebrae. The latter are often restricted and their stretching is not always sufficient. A direct action thrust of these structures may be required to release posterior peritoneal restrictions.

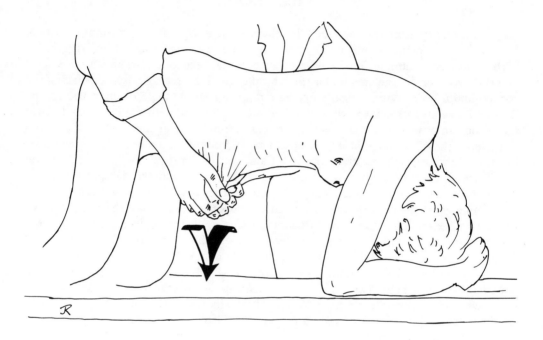

Illustration 2-4
Peritoneal Stretching (Knee/Elbow Position)

Recommendations

I urge you to always remain aware of the important mechanical role of the peritoneum. A peritoneal restriction will disturb the cohesion and functioning of the abdominal organs. Even expert manipulation of the cecum without release of the peritoneum does not bring significant results! Finish your treatment with induction techniques. Remember the general rule for induction, i.e., in the beginning you follow or go toward the restriction; as the restriction releases you progressively go away from it; at the end the release is complete and the movement stops.

Chapter Three:
The Gastroesophageal Junction

Table of Contents

The Gastroesophageal Junction

Physiology and Anatomy

The gastroesophageal junction and the bladder are the areas most subject to mechanical stresses, because both are located at zones of conflicting changes in pressure. The gastroesophageal junction is located where the thorax meets the abdomen, and the bladder where the abdomen meets the pelvis.

Intrathoracic pressure is negative (about $-5\,cm\,H_2O$) to allow pulmonary expansion. Intraabdominal pressure is positive (about $+5$ to $+10\,cm\,H_2O$). These two zones of opposing pressures are separated by the diaphragm, which contains several openings. The esophageal opening is surrounded by muscular and fibrous connective tissue, and can vary in diameter depending on respiratory and digestive activity. This opening must allow liquids and solids to pass into the stomach but prevent anything from returning into the esophagus; it is particularly important in preventing reflux of gastric secretions (esophageal reflux).

The gastroesophageal junction functions as a sphincter (I often refer to it as the "lower esophageal sphincter"), although technically it is not. It is an area of high pressure (between $+5$ and $10\,cm\,H_2O$) compared to that within the stomach. It relaxes on swallowing before the esophageal peristaltic wave arrives, and remains closed during the night. Numerous factors (to be discussed) may interfere with its optimal functioning.

The diaphragm is in permanent motion and its esophageal opening must function while following this motion. This increases the forces that result from opposing pressures. With even slight changes of tone, elasticity or extensibility of the fibromuscular system in this area, esophageal tissues are stretched and worn away because of diaphragmatic pounding. In acute periods they will be inflamed and irritated; when healed they will be fibrous and sclerosed. As a result, the shock-absorbing and occlusive functions of the gastroesophageal junction are impaired and malfunctions or illnesses (described below) develop. In order to clearly visualize the mobility of this junction, it is necessary to understand that in inhalation it is intraabdominal and in exhalation it is intrathoracic.

The gastroesophageal junction is an anatomical and physiological entity. Its proper function requires good tone and elasticity of the muscular fibers of the esophagus and of the cardia (upper part of the stomach), and that the cardia be neither too dilated nor too contracted. The junction should not suffer abnormal constraints from its anatomical environment, which includes the heart, mediastinum, pleura, lungs, diaphragm, liver (spigelian lobe), gastric fundus, peritoneum, vertebral column, and ribs. Opening and closing of the junction are associated with clockwise and counterclockwise (respectively) rotation of the esophagus, viewed from above.

During dissections I have had the opportunity to see many types of connections between the mediastinal area and the gastroesophageal junction. The majority of autopsies were of subjects who had suffered from tuberculosis or other serious pulmonary illnesses. The junction exchanges fibers with the pleura and the mediastinum; when scar tissue is present, the anatomical harmony of the area is disrupted. Next to the junction is found the left triangular ligament of the liver, which can become fibrosed following hepatitis. In *Visceral Manipulation*, we described the incessant hammering action of the diaphragm and, to a lesser extent, of the heart. Restrictions in this area lead to problems with elasticity and distensibility and, as a result, structural lesions.

As it passes through the diaphragmatic opening, the abdominal esophagus is accompanied by the vagus nerves (left anterior and right posterior). A mechanical disturbance may cause pulling on these nerves and consequent serious vagal problems, which I will discuss later. Surgeons take great care when approaching this area because of the richness of the nerve supply here. The celiac plexus is very close (posterior and to the right) to the cardia.

Pathology

The forces of negative intrathoracic pressure attract the diaphragmatic region and the organs which hang from it. When the mechanical harmony of the gastroesophageal junction is broken, it is always the stomach which migrates toward the esophagus, and not the opposite. With certain ruptures or hernias of the anterior fibrous part of the diaphragm, the splenic flexure of the colon may enter the thorax (I have actually seen this). Pierre Mercier, my colleague, brought me a case of a migration of part of the pancreas into the thorax, another example of the strength of the forces in this area.

For normal functioning of the gastroesophageal junction, the following general elements must be present:

- elastic and tonic diaphragm
- good longitudinal tension of the esophagus
- supple and distensible tissues which indirectly affect the junction (e.g., the psoas muscles via the diaphragm)
- a balance between thoracic and abdominal pressures
- good general condition of the body.

There are other more specific requirements. The angle of the cardiac notch must be acute. This angle is reinforced by a fold of the mucosa. The stomach's air pocket contributes to the formation of the cardiac notch, the gastric fundus being found higher

in the cardia. The portion of the diaphragm which forms the fibrous ring around the esophageal opening must have good tone and elasticity. The lining of the subdiaphragmatic
aponeurosis, which anchors the esophageal base, must be intact. The existence of pressure
which compresses the portion of the diaphragm below the junction is necessary in order
that the anatomical boundary between esophagus and stomach be maintained. This
phenomenon (pressure reinforcing a sphincter-like function) is reminiscent of the pelvic
manometric enclosure of the bladder.

When these conditions are not met, a hiatal hernia or esophageal reflux (discussed
below) may occur.

HIATAL HERNIA

Normally, the entire stomach is inferior to the diaphragm *(Illustration 3-1)*. In a
hiatal hernia, some portion of the stomach passes into the thorax through the esophageal
opening of the diaphragm. These hernias may be divided into sliding and unfolding types.

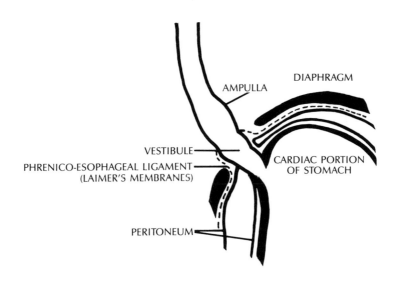

Illustration 3-1
Diaphragmatic Hiatus (Normal Relationships)

The sliding (or esophageal) type *(Illustration 3-2a)* is the most common. In this
type, the stomach and gastroesophageal junction migrate together into the thorax,
sometimes to such an extent that they are found above the diaphragmatic opening. On
radiography, the esophagus seems to be shortened, the gastroesophageal junction being
found in the thorax where abdominal pressures cannot reinforce it. In the unfolding
(or periesophageal) type of hernia *(Illustration 3-2b)*, the cardia of the stomach passes
through the diaphragmatic opening next to the gastroesophageal junction. This type of
hernia is seen mostly in women. There can also be mixed hernias.

I have treated numerous patients who presented the symptoms of a hiatal hernia but without radiological confirmation. This situation may result from a spasm of the gastroesophageal junction or abnormal tension of the surrounding tissues, i.e., abnormal elasticity or distensibility of fibrous connective tissues, or disturbed tonus of muscular tissues. Consider the example of a spasm of the left hemidiaphragm due to too large a pocket of air in the stomach, or a restriction of the left sixth costovertebral articulation. These both present functional mechanical problems similar to those of a hiatal hernia; the diagnosis can only be made by osteopathic means.

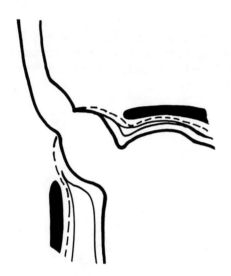
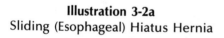
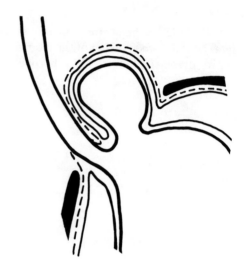

Illustration 3-2a
Sliding (Esophageal) Hiatus Hernia

Illustration 3-2b
Unfolding (Pariesophageal) Hiatus Hernia

Clinical Signs

A frequent manifestation of hiatal hernias, especially the sliding type, is esophageal reflux (see below). Unfortunately, one cannot distinguish between hiatal hernia and simple esophageal reflux by using listening. Among the symptoms of esophageal reflux caused by hiatal hernia are the following:

- pyrosis ('heartburn')
- regurgitation, belching, dysphagia
- epigastric or retrosternal pain worsened by certain movements, e.g., leaning forward
- stomach pain, watery and stringy vomiting, acidic breath
- lower chest pain
- pain which is increased by coughing and enforced exhalation
- pain accompanying eating
- headaches which are often relieved by vomiting.

ESOPHAGEAL REFLUX

I should note that a minor physiological esophageal reflux may exist normally when the gastroesophageal junction relaxes during sleep or after eating. This type is quickly overcome by esophageal peristalsis (which counters the reflux action), and saliva (which neutralizes the residual acid).

Other types of reflux are of more concern. The gastroesophageal junction needs good neurohormonal control and a good anatomical environment. There are several possible mechanisms for reflux. Periods of chaotic relaxation of muscle tissue around the gastroesophageal junction interfere with its sphincter-like function. Pressure within the stomach may exert too strong an effect on a hypotonic sphincter. Any abnormality of the mechanical pressures around the sphincter can also disturb its functioning. Muscular alterations can occur with scleroderma or following surgery. Any thoracic or abdominal surgery can affect the gastroesophageal junction because of the imbalance of reciprocal pressures involved. In a similar manner, one often finds inguinal hernias after seemingly benign surgery because the fibers of the rectus abdominis have had their normal interaction disrupted. However, when I mention muscular alteration in this chapter, I am referring to results of surgery on the esophagus or gastroesophageal junction.

Mechanisms of reflux involving "bad anatomical disposition" include a sliding hiatal hernia where the gastroesophageal junction is found in the thorax and abdominal pressure no longer reinforces it. A sliding hiatal hernia is the obvious example, but the slightest abnormality of tissues around the gastroesophageal junction can disturb it.

Neurohormonal alterations have an effect on the whole basic tone of the gastro-esophageal junction. Common causative states are depression and pregnancy. Other circumstances which alter this tone are certain drugs (e.g., oral contraceptives, antidepressants, tranquilizers, sedatives), foods (e.g., chocolate, citrus fruits, coffee, cigarettes, wine, sulfites), and restrictions which affect transmission of nerve impulses into and away from this area. Esophageal reflux associated with pregnancy is well known, and is often attributed to an increase in abdominal pressure. However, a more likely explanation may be a hormonal inhibition of sphincter-like function, analogous to stress incontinence of pregnancy.

Poor esophageal clearance is another possible mechanism. In all disorders involving alteration of the esophageal mucus (esophagitis, esophageal sclerosis, scleroderma, fibrous periesophageal tissues, idiopathic megaesophagus, etc.), clearance is abnormal. The gastroesophageal junction, as well as the esophagus itself, can be affected in this way.

With esophageal reflux, the pressure of the gastroesophageal junction is usually normal. This demonstrates that the cause of the problem must be somewhere else. Problems with neighboring organs may also produce reflux. When the stomach is prolapsed or fixed by adhesions, e.g. as the result of an ulcer, its attachments are strained. Stretching, particularly at the level of the gastrophrenic ligament and upper fundus, creates abnormal tensions of the cholinergic gastric fibers and vagus nerves. The gastroesophageal junction is thereby mechanically restricted and secretion of gastric acid increases, two conditions which can favor esophageal reflux. Other organs can pull the vagus nerves; e.g., the left extremity of the liver, or the membrane systems of the lungs and heart. Restrictions of L1-L2 are often found with abnormal anatomical tensions of the gastroesophageal junction.

Symptoms

Pyrosis (heartburn) is the major digestive symptom of esophageal reflux. Regurgitation of food or stomach acid is often associated with a burning sensation starting below the xiphoid process and extending up behind the sternum. These symptoms are exaggerated by bending forward or by wearing tight belts or clothing which cause abdominal compression. Pyrosis is commonly found in pregnancy because of abdominal compression and hormonally-induced hypotonus of the sphincter (see above), and often increases after meals. Patients may incorrectly call this reflux burning sensation a "gastritis." Reflux may also cause indigestion and increased saliva production, perhaps because of vagal excitation and a physiological attempt to neutralize esophageal irritation. Patients suffering from pyrosis do not like sour foods (especially at the end of the meal), and are attracted to sweets. The breath is often acidic. Esophageal reflux often causes a spasm of the gastroesophageal junction and the diaphragm.

There are a variety of other symptoms without obvious relationship to the digestive system. They include: morning pharyngeal irritation and dryness; ear pain resulting from inflammation of the auditory canal; sensitivity of the left side of the face; nocturnal and postprandial coughing; and bronchitic, asthmatic-type attacks occurring mostly during periods of maximal nocturnal vagal activity (2 to 4 A.M.). The latter symptom results not only from acid irritation of the bronchi, but also from bronchoconstriction of vagal origin. These asthmatic-type attacks can also occur after an abnormally large meal or one eaten too quickly. This perhaps explains some good results which certain people attribute too readily to treatment of true asthma due to sensitivity or other problems of the bronchioles.

Other symptoms include pseudo-angina (these lower chest pains are of vagal origin or possibly a symptom of esophageal irritation) and cardiorespiratory distress in the newborn. The latter was described in 1986 by Professor Charpoy of Marseille (Symposium des Ormeaux at the Le Havre). Esophageal reflux in infants is more often related to neurological maturation than to somatic development. That is, neurological maturation of the gastroesophageal junction is completed very late in intrauterine development. In the postpartum period, the sphincter may take six to eight weeks to become fully functional. Before the age of fifteen months, reflux is manifested primarily as digestive problems; after that time respiratory problems surface.

Regurgitation is the rejection of esophageal or gastric contents, via the mouth, without particular effort or discomfort. It is not the same as esophageal reflux nor is it necessarily a sign of that condition. It is sometimes seen as early morning vomiting in alcoholics. Everyone, at some time, may have experienced regurgitation, often after breakfast. It is a common phenomenon which, typically, is due to the stomach having difficulties adapting to a large quantity of liquid.

Chronic esophageal reflux may result in peptic esophagitis, in which the lining of the esophagus is slowly destroyed. In this condition, the normal lining of the esophagus is replaced by sclerosed scar tissue to the point where stenoses result.

Dysphagia (difficulty in swallowing) after ingestion of solids, and especially liquids, can be a warning sign of cancer. There is a risk of cancer developing with chronic esophageal lesions. If there is any possibility of this, don't hesitate to obtain a radiographic or endoscopic exam.

Etiology

Hiatal hernia and esophageal reflux do not always occur together. However, they do share similar predisposing factors. One important cause is loosening of connective tissues and loss of basic tonus with increasing age. Age *per se* is probably not the causative factor; these conditions are typically seen in patients between 35 and 50 years of age, and to me seem to be correlated with hormonal cycles. With acquired thoracic kyphosis, there is a change in the relationship between the gastroesophageal junction and the diaphragm, reducing the efficiency of the sphincter-like function.

Depression and other general disorders which affect the general tonus of the patient can be a factor in hypotonus of the gastroesophageal junction. Unusual efforts (coughing, sneezing, defecation, expectoration) which provoke significant rises in abdominal pressure (50 to 100cm H_2O) can irritate and injure the junction and its attachments.

Menopause and the male climacteric are periods of hormonal imbalance in which problems often occur. There are also other cycles, such as the changes that occur with the seasons, or changes in testosterone levels which occur in the late 30s. Clinically, these cycles seem to be associated with development of reflux, but the mechanisms are not clear.

Surgery results in imbalanced tensions in all tissues associated with the scars. Certain occupations (besides the classic example of the pneumatic drill operator) can contribute to destabilization of the gastroesophageal junction, e.g., activities such as painting which necessitate raising the arms in the air. Sedentary work, particularly the vibrations associated with frequent traveling, contributes to loosening of the gastroesophageal junction attachments. Finally, a certain category of patients seems to be predisposed toward this type of pathology, for no obvious reason. Do they suffer from a congenital or hereditary malposition of the gastroesophageal junction?

Osteopaths know that asymptomatic restrictions can create lesions at a distance. Thus, restrictions of the diaphragmatic crura can affect the gastroesophageal junction. In fact, it is my experience that when there are upper lumbar restrictions in patients with problems of the gastroesophageal junction, therapeutic results will be better (when mobilization of those restrictions is included in the treatment) than with such patients without upper lumbar restrictions.

Cranial trauma can also have repercussions on the gastroesophageal junction, through abnormal stimulation of the vagal nerves as they exit through the jugular foramen. I have no objective proof of this etiology but the clinical facts speak for themselves. Still, the successes which I have had utilizing cranial manipulation with newborn infants should be interpreted with caution; sometimes the problem is a neurological immaturity of the gastroesophageal junction which resolves itself in time. Does manipulation merely accompany a favorable evolution, or does it accelerate it?

Letting a hernia evolve by itself can sometimes cause serious risks. Surgical intervention may be necessary in cases of obstruction, perforation, strangulation, and hemorrhage. However, surgery should be avoided whenever possible and gentler techniques used instead.

OTHER DISORDERS

At the beginning of this section, I wish to emphasize the care and reserve which a practitioner should always use in the presence of a pathology which may appear to be routine. As the reader has observed, disorders ranging from the trivial to the life-threatening may share similar symptoms.

Cardiospasm refers to disordered motor function of the distal esophagus and failure of the gastric cardia to relax. This can lead to esophageal reflux because of abnormal tension of the cardia as well as the esophagus. Peristalsis is disrupted and the junction shortens. Subsequently, normal peristaltic contractions are replaced by disorderly stationary contractions and the junction does not shorten any more, reflecting a change in the esophagus' cholinergic innervation. One notices a rarefaction of Meissner's and Auerbach's plexuses. The stasis and dilatation of the esophagus result in its abnormal enlargement.

In *cardioesophageal laceration (Mallory-Weiss syndrome)*, the mucosa of the gastroesophageal junction is longitudinally torn, a laceration which is accompanied by massive hemorrhage. This syndrome can be found after any process that adversely affects the gastroesophageal junction, e.g., vomiting, coughing, childbirth, difficult defecation, thoracic trauma, alcoholism, hiatal hernia, and surgery in the area of the esophagus.

Esophageal perforations, which occur following intense coughing or vomiting, shock, or infection, are characterized by intense pain, air in the mediastinum accompanied by subcutaneous emphysema, and respiratory complications such as hemopneumothorax. The mediastinal pleura is attacked or even digested by the gastric juices. The results of these perforations indicate the significance of the pressures in this area.

Subphrenic abscess is characterized by retroscapular pain, abdominal pain, uncontrollable hiccoughing episodes, bronchial congestion, and fever.

Cruveilhier-Baumgarten syndrome is characterized by a very dilated paraumbilical venous system (like a medusa's head), portal hypertension, liver atrophy, splenomegaly, and varicose veins of the esophagus and cardia. These phenomena appear when stasis of the portal vein causes part of the venous blood to use the portal-cava anastomosis, leading to esophageal varicose veins and hemorrhoids. This syndrome is found with advanced age, pregnancy, depression, weight loss, liver problems, general fatigue, overeating, alcoholism, and unfavorable work positions.

Esophageal cancer is the fifth most common cancer in adult males, who are at greater risk than females. Symptoms include: progressive dysphagia that begins with solid foods and gradually progresses to include semisolid foods and finally liquids; anorexia; significant weight loss over a short period of time; retrosternal, thoracic and cervical pain; retrosternal burning sensations after ingestion of hot drinks; blood-stained regurgitations; lymph node metastasis, particularly in the left supraclavicular fossa (known as a signal node or Virchow's node); and subcutaneous emphysema of the neck from mediastinitis.

Be very alert to any of the above conditions (except cardiospasm). They are absolute contraindications for direct manipulation of this area because of the risk of overwhelming hemorrhage.

In conclusion, most common disorders of the gastroesophageal junction are structural in origin. Osteopaths, of course, delight in structural lesions as we are most effective in treating them. You must check thoroughly for lesions of the junction itself, as well as neighboring structures. Your actions and degree of success will depend on the extent to which the tissues are fibrous. The more fibrous the tissues, the more structure you have to work with and therefore successful manipulation will lead to more dramatically significant changes.

Diagnosis

In terms of general listening, it is difficult to differentiate problems of the gastroesophageal junction from those of the stomach. In both situations, the patient bends directly forward and then gently rotates to the left. With problems of the gastroesophageal junction, forward bending is more pronounced than it is for the stomach.

For local differential diagnosis of the gastroesophageal junction, place your hand on the patient's abdomen with the middle finger along the midline, heel on the umbilicus, and fingers slightly spread. The middle finger is pulled toward the xiphoid process and, gradually, the palm also moves up. The palm is then pulled backward, toward the vertebral column (T11) and very slightly to the left (the cardia is found a little to the left of the median line). At the end of the process the palm is flattened against and compresses the xiphoid process.

For diagnosis of the celiac plexus, the palm remains slightly inferior and to the right of the xiphoid process and rocks either antero-posteriorly or from side to side. Celiac plexus problems are marked by superficial emotional problems or vagal dysfunction. For the liver, the middle finger is drawn to the right and the palm contacts the lower right costal margin. For the stomach, the middle finger moves to the left of the midline, and the palm is found between the umbilicus and the lower left costal margin.

Differential diagnosis is difficult with injuries to the lower parts of the pulmonary area. The palm does not stay against the xiphoid process but tends to move above it. With lateral pulmonary injury, the diagnosis is easier; the hand moves unmistakably onto the thorax. For the esophagus, the hand is attracted by and goes past the xiphoid process. At the same time, the hand is not pulled as deeply posterior as when listening to the gastroesophageal junction.

DIAGNOSTIC MANIPULATION

In the presence of a hiatal hernia, pain in the area of the cardia increases with exhalation. With exhalation, the gastroesophageal junction is already in an intrathoracic position and forced exhalation increases its thoracic penetration, causing the pain sensation. However, forced inhalation also creates pain by forcing the supporting tissues of the junction to lengthen. During inhalation, the patient will stop before the end of the movement in order to prevent this stretching. Coughing and sneezing, as well as visceral manipulation causing the abdomen to move during periods when the diaphragm is still, will also stimulate this area and cause pain.

Aggravation/Relief

For hiatal hernia, an aggravation technique can be performed with the patient in the seated position. Place yourself behind the patient and place your fingers slightly below and to the left of the xiphoid, and then move them in deeply as if you wished to reach the vertebral column *(Illustration 3-3)*. The more the patient leans forward, the easier it is to go in deeply because of the relaxation of the rectus abdominis muscle, peritoneum, greater omentum and stomach. At maximum penetration, without the technique being painful, bring the fingers superiorly and slightly to the right. The stomach is thus pushed posterosuperiorly (this has been verified by fluoroscopy). In the case of a hiatal hernia, you will immediately set off a sensation of retroxiphoidal pain comparable to that which the patient knows. This pain is often accompanied by nausea and a distinct malaise. To further aggravate the problem, ask the patient to exhale deeply at the end of the technique.

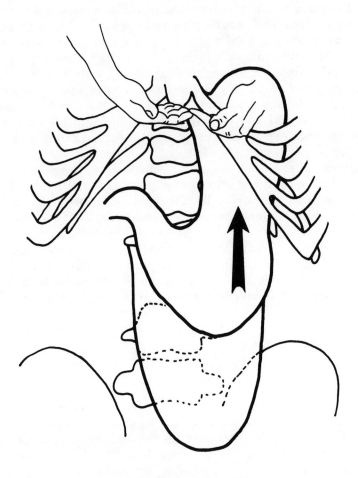

Illustration 3-3
Aggravation Technique

At the end of the aggravation technique, quickly release the pressure (recoil technique). If the patient feels a deep irritation, it means that the gastroesophageal junction and surrounding tissues are irritated, and probably fibrosed. If pain is felt during manipulation, it means that the stomach itself is irritated. Alternatively, press strongly on the left 11th costovertebral articulation or the posterior angle of R11 on the left. When there is irritation of the cardia, you will increase the malaise or pain that the patient is feeling. This technique can be performed in isolation or actively accompanying inhalation.

The relief technique *(Illustration 3-4)* is performed in the seated position with the fingers subcostal, as with the aggravation technique. Move the abdominal fingers anteroinferiorly so as to relax the pressure of the gastroesophageal junction in the thorax. If the patient feels relief, this suggests a problem involving the gastroesophageal junction.

A diminution or accentuation of the symptoms in this manner supports the diagnosis of a mechanical lesion of the gastroesophageal junction. However, this cannot eliminate the possibility of a more serious pathology.

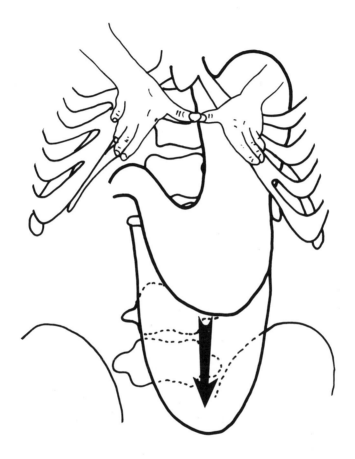

Illustration 3-4
Relief Technique

ASSOCIATED SKELETAL RESTRICTIONS

Restrictions of the cervical column frequently accompany problems of the gastroesophageal junction. Restrictions are a little more common on the left, accompanied by those of the sternoclavicular joint, and may reflect abnormal tension of the fasciae which join the cervical column and gastroesophageal junction, or alternatively irritation of the vagus and phrenic nerves.

Restrictions of the thoracic vertebrae and ribs may also be involved. The 11th left costovertebral articulation, and R7 on the left, correspond to the posterior and anterior anatomical projections of the cardia respectively. Sensitivity or pain upon palpation of the 7th costochondral articulation suggests restriction of the cardia.

T12, L1, L2, L3 can become fixed because of mechanical irritation and correspond to the diaphragmatic crura. These restrictions are more serious when on the left and decrease the mobility of the left hemidiaphragm, as you can see when watching the patient breathe. These reflex restrictions of thoracic vertebrae produce sensitivity but not complete loss of mobility. In such cases, backward bending causes retroxiphoidal pain through stretching of the gastroesophageal junction. The patient often reacts by holding his breath. Forward bending will immediately stop this type of pain.

The gastroesophageal junction may also affect certain parts of the body that are known to become restricted for a wide variety of reasons. For example, the left sacroiliac articulation may become restricted secondarily to problems in many other areas, and for this reason is sometimes referred to as the body's "waste basket." Similarly, the psoas muscles are often involved in various disorders, but are seldom a cause themselves. The left psoas is often spasmed in patients with gastroesophageal problems, in part because its attachments exchange fibers with the diaphragm. The sympathetic nerves which traverse it can also become irritated in this situation.

OTHER DIAGNOSTIC CONSIDERATIONS

Patients with problems of the gastroesophageal junction have a tendency to stand bent forward with the right shoulder slightly forward, and the left shoulder back and lowered. The slight left rotation seems to result from the cardia bending obliquely at the bottom on the left.

Perhaps because of the involvement of the vagus and phrenic nerves, the Adson-Wright test is usually positive on the left when there are problems of the gastroesophageal junction. It is instructive to perform an Adson-Wright test while also performing a relief movement. Take the pulse in one hand, and with the other create a compression/inhibition point of the anterior projection of the cardia, toward the 7th costochondral cartilage. With a mechanical problem of the gastroesophageal junction, this technique will cause the radial pulse to quickly improve or return. With a hiatal hernia, the cervical/thoracic fasciae are often more tense on the left. These tensions can also render the Adson-Wright test positive. Left systolic pressure is sometimes lower, but this is more rare than with problems of the stomach itself.

Problems of the gastroesophageal junction can produce many other distant symptoms. Left cervical neck pain and cervical/brachial neuralgia may occur, due to irritation of the cervical/brachial plexuses provoked by the phrenic nerve and excessive tension of the cervical fasciae. The 4th left costochondral space is often sensitive. This is manifested in women as mammary pain and in men as lower chest pain. For the same reason as with neck pain, glenohumeral periarthritis may be found on the left. You can perform a glenohumeral test using one hand to test the left shoulder and the other to inhibit the anterior projection of the cardia, or by using a relief movement.

The most common cranial lesions related to gastroesophageal dysfunction are found at the level of the left temporomandibular joint, left occipitomastoid suture and, in newborns, the jugular foramen. As mentioned above, neurological maturation of the gastroesophageal junction in infants takes place gradually, and esophageal reflux generally resolves over time.

A hiatal hernia can be responsible for vagal irritations which can cause a feeling of faintness or even brief loss of consciousness, and associated symptoms of indigestion.

Lower chest pain is also of vagal origin. You may treat patients (usually men) who have the disagreeable sensation of "feeling their heart" and sometimes an electric, dagger-thrust type of tearing sensation in the chest. Such patients may be convinced that they suffer from a heart disease, and request various cardiological examinations, which are all negative. They may then have their symptoms labeled as 'psychosomatic' and feel abandoned. We all know how worrying it is to feel cardiac pain. Stretching of the vagus nerve can irritate the heart, and chest pain is almost always accompanied by a restriction of the 4th left costochondral articulation. This type of restriction is rare in real cardiac problems, while restrictions of T4 itself are relatively common.

Treatment

The purpose of treatment is to reinforce and relax the gastroesophageal junction by induction focused on this area, and to free any fibromuscular restrictions of the junction and surrounding structures.

DIRECT TECHNIQUE

Place the patient in the seated position, hands behind the base of the neck with fingers interlaced. At the beginning, this is the same position as for the relief technique

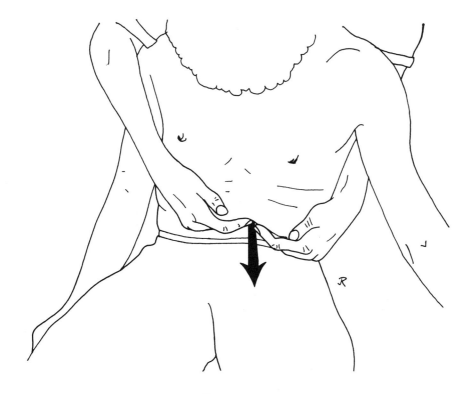

Illustration 3-5
Local Direct Technique

described above. Place your fingers 3-4 cm under the xiphoid process and slightly to the left of the midline. Delicately and progressively push the fingers inward past the liver until you reach the limit of discomfort. Gently relax the pressure so as not to create a guarding reflex. If you cannot reach the liver, get as close as you can. Leave your left hand in place, using it as an anchor point for the stomach. With your right hand, backward bend the patient by using the elbows. The distance from the xiphoid to the umbilicus is thus increased and the stomach is pulled downward, lowering the cardia and pulling the gastroesophageal junction out of the thorax.

Repeat this technique 5-6 times until pain is reduced. In a few sessions, the tissues of the gastroesophageal junction will recover their natural distensibility. Since the cardia faces downward and to the left, stretching of the thorax upward and to the right will increase the efficiency of the technique.

A variation of this technique is performed in the same position *(Illustration 3-5)*. Place both hands in the abdominal position and apply movements of the fingers downward and slightly anteriorly. Move the fingers from top to bottom to reach the areas (there are usually three or four) which feel tight. With thin and supple patients you can perform this technique with the fingers very high up, underneath the left extremity of the liver (which is anterior to the stomach), against the gastroesophageal junction.

RECOIL

A hepatic recoil technique is very helpful in treating gastroesophageal restrictions. It is also performed in the seated position. Establish a pressure point under the liver, with the two hands near the attachments of the left and right triangular ligaments. Push the liver posterosuperiorly, release it quickly, and repeat the movement 3-4 times. Initially, this movement will be painful as it goes toward the lesion, but the pain will progressively disappear. This very effective technique frees the connective fibers around the gastroesophageal junction which affect the liver.

INDUCTION

For an induction technique of the cardia, place the patient in the seated position. Put one hand posteriorly at the level of the 11th left costovertebral articulation, and the other anteriorly on the 7th left costochondral cartilage. Initially, the anterior hand presses on the thorax in the direction of the posterior hand, and both hands move slightly inferiorly. Sometimes there are also slight lateral movements. The hands work in concert and, as the tissues begin to release, you will feel a separation between the hands, signaling the end of manipulation. This technique has a passive aspect (the induction consists of following the tissues), but you also move your hands actively toward the cardia. The technique seems to act above all on spasms of the gastroesophageal junction and is a very powerful treatment for all the attachments in the area (including those of the pericardium, pleura, stomach and liver). You can also perform this technique with the patient in the supine position, which is less work for you but not quite as effective, since the pull of gravity toward the feet is not utilized.

Recommendations

When dealing with a particularly fibrosed gastroesophageal junction which is limited by the left hemidiaphragm, try stretching the psoas. Such stretching has a pronounced effect on a hiatal hernia. There are many effective ways to stretch the psoas. I prefer either the prone or lateral recumbent position, where one hand stabilizes the sacrum and pelvis while the other extends the thigh.

For greatest effectiveness, these techniques must be performed in a specific order:

- Free the areas of attachment of the liver
- Free the pylorus and the stomach (fundal area)
- Free the gastroesophageal junction
- Manipulate important skeletal restrictions which persist, particularly those of the costochondral articulations
- Use the induction technique described above
- Normalize cranial restrictions.

This sequence allows the successive elimination of all vertebral and cranial restrictions which are reflex in nature, and enables you to concentrate on those which are most primary.

Beware of these symptoms: rapid weight loss, dysphagia, blood-stained regurgitation, left supraclavicular nodes, or subcutaneous emphysema. Any of these may indicate malignancy or some other serious condition.

ADVICE TO THE PATIENT

In cases of hiatal hernia or esophageal reflux, the patient should be advised as follows:

- Do not go to sleep immediately after a meal
- Do not wear tight belts or clothing
- Sleep on a fairly high pillow
- Avoid staying in a forward bending or reverse Trendelenburg position
- Sleep with the head and upper thorax on a pillow
- Do not hold the arms in the air and head tilted back for a long time
- When straining, try to hold onto the lower part of the ribs with the hands
- Avoid constipation. Be careful about ingestion of oranges, chocolate, coffee, tea, alcohol, fats, vinegar, mustard and tobacco.

These foods may, however, be well tolerated depending upon the hour of ingestion. For example, oranges are better tolerated at the beginning of a meal. Chocolate and alcohol should be especially avoided in the evening before going to bed. Other foods may be toxic in specific combinations or depending on specific physiological conditions. Female patients should avoid all these foodstuffs just before menstruation, because of the hormonal effects on the gastroesophageal junction.

Chapter Four:
The Stomach and Duodenum

Table of Contents

The Stomach and Duodenum

I have separated the discussion of the stomach from that of the gastroesophageal junction purely for didactic reasons. The cardia and gastric fundus are integral parts of the stomach. Naturally, their mechanical conflicts (see chapter 3) are also applicable to this chapter.

Physiology and Anatomy

The stomach is drawn toward the diaphragm as if by a magnet and is flattened underneath it. Forces associated with respiration pull the fibers of the cardia, cardiac notch, and gastric fundus upward and slightly toward the back. The stomach's superior attachment system is essentially represented by the gastrophrenic ligament which is often overutilized and becomes fibrosed, thereby exerting too great a tension on the gastric mucosa and muscles into which it is inserted.

Pressure immediately below the diaphragm is around $-5\,cm\,H_2O$, but increases rapidly toward the central abdomen, up to $+10\,cm$ near the umbilicus. Thus, within a few centimeters, the pressures exerted on the stomach are reversed. If the superior attachments and the portion of the stomach next to the diaphragm become irritated, swollen, etc., transmission of these pressures via the diaphragm is disturbed. The negative pressures adjacent to the diaphragm become positive and mechanical conflicts inevitably result.

The stomach is contiguous with the left hemidiaphragm, which is more fibrous anteriorly and receives most of its innervation from the phrenic nerve, which also receives sensory information from the peritoneum to which it is attached.

The stomach leaves a large impression on the left lobe of the liver, both organs being connected by the lesser omentum. Because of this interdependence, the two organs must always be considered together in diagnosis and treatment.

Via the diaphragm, the stomach has a relationship with the heart and its coverings, as shown by the common occurrence of lower chest pain originating with the stomach but perceived near the heart. The lungs and pleurae are also attached to the diaphragm. Thus, pulmonary pathologies can affect the stomach via the diaphragm.

The area where the anterior surface of the stomach is in direct contact with the anterior abdominal wall is called Labbe's triangle. This triangle is bounded inferiorly by a horizontal line through the lower edge of the cartilage of R9, laterally by the costal margin, and on the right by the liver. Listening usually takes place between the liver and the left costal margin. Traube's semilunar space is found in the left anterior part of the lower thorax. This space is bounded medially by the left side of the sternum, superiorly by an oblique line going from the sixth costal cartilage to the lower aspect of R8-9, and inferiorly by the costal margin. In this space there are no vibrations which can be felt with palpation, and respiratory noises can be heard with auscultation.

Restrictions of the costovertebral articulations are pathogenic for the stomach. Manipulation of the stomach without adjustment of such restrictions is not a complete treatment. Osteopaths are always conscious of vertebral articulations but often forget the costovertebral articulations, which, in my opinion, are equally (or possibly more) important. As with the other viscera, dysfunctions of many distant parts of the body may affect the stomach. Specifically, the clavicle and the first and second sternocostal articulations are often involved.

The stomach is protected against chemical, mechanical and (particularly) thermal damage by a mucous membrane. For example, most people are able to drink coffee at temperatures of 50-70°C, more than the maximum temperature that the skin can support. Paradoxically, the stomach is better at withstanding this type of abuse than it is at handling stress-related reactions. It is likely to be irritated when acid and basic secretions are present simultaneously (or serially); ulcers are often found in these cases. When the stomach is distended, the pylorus secretes the hormone gastrin. Gastric evacuation increases when the ileum is active or externally stimulated, which allows us to utilize certain techniques applied to the ileum for treatment of the stomach.

The upper part of the stomach is cholinergic (i.e., stimulated by acetylcholine from autonomic nerve fibers). Mechanoreceptors in the stomach, when excited, release gastric secretions such as HCl which, in large quantities, can become toxic. Cholinergic reactions of the fundal area may be involved in some stomach pains and diseases of mechanical origin. Contrary to popular belief, practically no iron is absorbed in the stomach. However, HCl and an "intrinsic factor" secreted by the stomach lining are essential for absorption of vitamin B12, which is needed for red blood cell formation.

The pylorus prevents reflux into the stomach when the pressure in the superior duodenum increases, and brings large particles back toward the stomach for more mechanical digestion. When the pylorus is open (e.g., when the stomach is empty), it is located to the left of the midline; when the pylorus is contracted (or the person is nervous and tense), it is to the right. I believe that the pylorus, like the gastroesophageal junction, may act as a sphincter, although few gastroenterologists would agree with me. I must admit that, seen from the inside, it does not resemble a sphincter. During several experiments using fiber optics, I noticed that it is nearly always open. However, it is in fact a contractile muscular structure with a few circular fibers. If these remain contracted, they can cause pyloric spasms which can be easily felt externally. For this reason, I consider the pylorus as having sphincter-like reflexogenic properties.

When the pyloric area is mechanically distended or exposed to an alkaline solution, gastrin is secreted. Gastrin has the effect of increasing gastric acid and peptic secretions, gastric and intestinal motility, exogenous pancreatic secretions, biliary output, and tonus of the gastroesophageal junction.

Slight mechanical disturbances or spasms may cause major physiological disorders. Finding and treating a pyloric restriction sometimes gives us unexpectedly great results. Remember that 55 percent of duodenal contractions take place when the antral region contracts or is stimulated. This gives the pylorus a major influence on the duodenum. During digestion, the pylorus allows transit from the stomach to the duodenum approximately three times per minute.

Anatomy of the duodenum has been described previously *(Visceral Manipulation, pp. 141-143)*. The four portions of the duodenum, leading from the stomach to the large intestine, will be referred to here as the superior, descending, inferior, and ascending duodenum respectively.

Pathology

GENERAL SYMPTOMS

The most common general symptom of stomach and duodenal dysfunction is epigastric pain. This will be discussed at length below, in the sections on ulcer, cancer and prolapse. Here we will cover a number of systemic symptoms relating in various degrees to the stomach. They should be well understood before manipulation of the stomach is considered.

Aerophagy (swallowing of air), abdominal distention, and flatulence are symptoms (not diseases) accompanied by diverse indispositions. They may be associated with compulsive belching after swallowing air (also known as swallower's twitch), gastric atonia or hypotonia, or pyloric spasms. These symptoms may result from dyspepsia, prolapse, ulcer, neoplasms, etc., or disorders of other organs (e.g., cholecystitis, appendicitis, angina pectoris, hepatic insufficiency, etc.). One could even say that they exist with each of these illnesses and that you cannot use them as conclusive evidence to diagnose any one of them.

Vomiting

Vomiting caused by stomach pain immediately relieves that pain. It is often provoked in cases of hypersthenic or ulcerous stomach disorders, and is often acidic. For projectile vomiting without nausea, malaise, anxiety or faintness, one must consider direct stimulation from the medulla resulting from endocranial hypertension (tumor, abscess, meningitis, etc.). Aqueous vomiting, made up of nearly pure gastric juices, is very acidic and accompanied by intense pyrosis. It is found with hyperchlorhydria and ulcers with significant acid secretion. Mucous and stringy vomiting is the classic early morning vomiting of viscous secretions observed in alcoholic gastritis.

Odorless vomiting of intact food suggests an esophageal diverticulum. Vomiting of acidic and burning partially-digested food with a sour smell, on the other hand, suggests hyperchlorhydria. Delayed vomiting of little-digested food indicates a reduction in gastric juice secretion, whereby the bolus is inadequately digested. Very delayed vomiting involves remnants of food ingested one or more days before and suggests a stenotic disorder of the pylorus. Recent physiological studies show that food can take up to five days to pass through the digestive system.

Vomiting of bile is often found in gastric pathologies when the patient has already vomited his gastric contents, and thereafter vomits a green liquid which is made up of vesicular bile and then of hepatic bile which is pale yellow. With vomiting of blood, you must make the proper studies to be sure that it is of gastric (and not respiratory, esophageal or duodenal) origin.

Bleeding

A gastric ulcer involves abundant hemorrhaging of bright red, fresh blood. With a duodenal ulcer, there is hematemesis (vomiting of blood of all origins), always followed by a significant melena (anal evacuation of black blood, which looks like tar, mixed with the stools). With cancer, there are small repeated hemorrhages of black (occasionally red) blood which has been more or less digested. If melena is abundant, one must consider a pyloric or duodenal ulcer which evacuates by the intestinal route. Discrete or repeated melena suggests small hemorrhages from an ulcer. However, copious melena may reflect a neoplasm or, more rarely, gastritis resulting from a hiatal or diaphragmatic hernia.

ULCER

Gastric ulcer is less frequent than that of the duodenum and typically affects men between 45 and 55 years of age. It is found most commonly on the lesser curvature and the antrum, and results from some defect in gastric mucosal resistance, or mucosal injury. Symptoms include dyspepsia and postprandial nausea. The pain/feeding/relief cycle takes place but is much less predictable than in duodenal ulcer; often, eating actually increases the pain. There is also less nocturnal pain than with a duodenal ulcer. It is difficult to establish the diagnosis, and difficult to distinguish benign from precancerous ulcers, except by a combination of radiography and endoscopy.

Duodenal ulcers are a common affliction, found in 6-15% of the population in the United States and representing approximately 75% of all ulcers. It is slightly more common in males, and the incidence is highest for men in their late 30s and early 40s. This type of ulcer is usually found in the transition zones between the fundal/antral or antral/duodenal mucosa. In one-third of the cases, duodenal ulcers are associated with gastric ulcers. Acid secretion is more abundant than with a gastric ulcer (men secrete more than women), and diminishes after 50 years of age, which explains why this disorder is more common in the younger age groups.

Causes include hypersecretion of gastric juices (notably during nocturnal vagal activity); genetic, emotional and endocrine factors (hyperparathyroidism increases the chance of ulcer formation ten-fold); cirrhosis, pancreatitis, and chronic lung disorders; iatrogenic factors (e.g., use of anti-inflammatory drugs); pancreatic or duodenal reflux; costovertebral restrictions; and seasonal rhythms (equinoctial increases in pain are well known). There are also more curious rhythms. Often, for example, pain reappears every five years without apparent explanation. In my opinion, these phenomena underscore the importance of gastric dependence on the endocrine system.

Many ulcers, perhaps 20-30%, are asymptomatic. The most common symptom is epigastric pain that is burning or gnawing in nature (it can also be boring, aching or vague). Typically, the pain occurs 1.5 to 3 hours after eating and is relieved within a few minutes by ingestion of food. An exception to this is sugar, which often makes the pain worse, especially when eaten on an empty stomach. The pain frequently awakens the patient between 2 and 4 A.M., and occasionally occurs just before breakfast. The pain is usually on the midline and may radiate mildly to the right. These patients often experience regurgitation and frequent belching. Weight loss is rare because the patient eats a lot to alleviate the pain.

Major complications of a duodenal ulcer include perforation, which often happens on the anterior side of the duodenum. Pain is sudden, intense and continuous, and is epigastric or slightly to the right, with possible radiation to the clavicles. The stomach is immobile because of a defensive contraction. Abdominal palpation, therefore, is difficult or impossible. The rectal exam is painful as the gastric juices collect in Douglas' pouch. There is the possibility of confusion with appendicitis or peritonitis. In addition, an ulcer can cause hematemesis, melena, or fainting (which may signify the loss of 1-1.5 liters of blood). These symptoms occur in 20% of hemorrhage cases. This is one good reason for taking the patient's arterial pressure before manipulation. If systolic pressure is too low, always consider a bleeding ulcer.

An ulcer can sometimes be localized based on the area of projected pain, as follows *(Dousset, 1964):* epigastric (ulcer of the lesser curvature); xiphoidal (ulcer of the cardia); right subcostal (pyloric or duodenal ulcer); left subcostal (ulcer of the greater curvature or the pyloric antrum); thoracic or lumbar (posterior ulcer). This topography is not always accurate or reliable, but I do find it interesting.

Alternatively, the ulcer can be localized on the basis of time and circumstance, as follows: at the beginning of a meal (simple stomach pain or gastritis); cramps when fasting calmed by food intake (gastric hypersecretion); hunger pains calmed after a meal (pyloric or duodenal ulcer); pain 1-2 hours after the meal, calmed by food intake (hypochlorhydria with or without an ulcer); pain for 4 hours after the meal (low-placed ulcer, juxtapyloric or duodenal).

The general time of occurrence of the pain is also of diagnostic importance. Cyclical pain is usually from ulcers. In cases of pain occurring without any known precipitant and in no particular cycle, cancer must be considered and ruled out. Positional pain or that occurring after a hastily-eaten meal is often due to gastric prolapse. Reflex stomach pain, accompanying pain in other areas, is probably due to other pathologies such as those involving the gallbladder and pancreas.

CANCER

Gastric cancer is twice as frequent in men, especially those with type A blood. The prevalence of this disease, fortunately, is diminishing. Perhaps this is due to increasing use of refrigerators, which lessen the need for nitrosamines as food additives. Over 90% of gastric cancers are carcinomas, found most commonly in the antrum and lesser curvature of the stomach. Symptoms of gastric cancer are: anorexia with particular distaste for meat and fatty foods; weight loss, general fatigue, anemia, and yellowish complexion; abdominal malaise, diarrhea, and low grade fevers; hepatomegaly, nodular liver with parietal induration which adheres to neighboring formations; and enlargement of the left supraclavicular lymph nodes and left pectoral node. In my experience, any patient complaining of alternating diarrhea and constipation accompanied by epigastric pain should always be examined carefully for gastric cancer.

GASTRIC PROLAPSE

There are, essentially, two types of mechanical gastric pathology. The superior type involves the movement of part of the stomach into the diaphragmatic opening through which the esophagus passes (see chapter 3). The superoinferior type is illustrated in the case of a gastric prolapse. This is really more a case of excessive lengthening of the stomach than of a true prolapse, in which the fundus is no longer contiguous with the diaphragm (very rare). I use the term here because of its common usage. Traditional gastroenterologists do not generally consider gastric prolapses pathological. I believe that this view comes from paying insufficient attention to the functional aspects of the body. To be sure, some prolapses remain asymptomatic, but others produce obvious dysfunction, especially when gastric mobility is affected. I believe that the difference is in this mobility itself, i.e., prolapses without disturbance of mobility are often asymptomatic, while those with disturbance of mobility are likely to be pathological.

The upper part of the stomach is drawn upward by the diaphragm and the lower part downward by gravity *(Illustration 4-1)*. With age, the organs tend to slide downward; movement of even a few centimeters is enough to alter the pressures which affect the stomach.

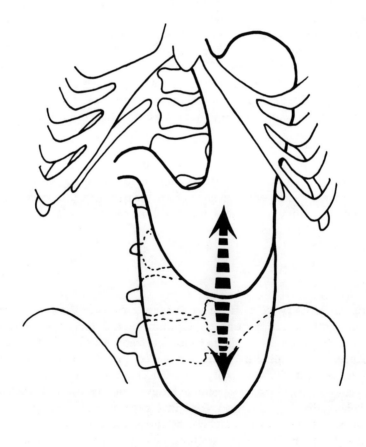

Illustration 4-1
Pressures on the Stomach

As noted (chapter 3), pressure adjacent to the diaphragm is negative (approximately $-5 \text{cm H}_2\text{O}$), but increases quickly to $+5$ to $10 \text{cm H}_2\text{O}$ in the superior fundal region and $+10$ to $15 \text{cm H}_2\text{O}$ at the level of the umbilicus. Pressures may increase further below the umbilicus, from $+20$ to $30 \text{cm H}_2\text{O}$ at the junction of the abdomen and pelvis. Clearly, the superior and inferior extremes of the stomach are subject to different pressures and mechanical restrictions. Movement of the inferior part downward, past its normal anatomical limits, results in stretching of all the mechanical structures which attach to it.

There are various causes of gastric prolapse. The tension of pleural and pulmonary tissues diminishes with age and disturbs the balance of abdominal pressures. The greater omentum and small intestine move gradually downward, pulling the stomach with them. This type of prolapse often involves the mesenteric root following a line going from the ileocecal junction to the umbilicus. Look carefully at your patients and you will note this phenomenon. With age, the tissues of the abdominal wall lose their tonicity, elasticity, and extensibility. Acquired kyphosis (exaggeration of the normal curve of the thoracic spine) can also contribute to gastric prolapse, in a manner analogous to that of a tie which moves down as you lean forward.

Pregnancy and childbirth are also frequent causes of gastric prolapse. Increases of abdominal pressure may be involved, but the major causes are hormonally-induced hypotonus of the supporting tissues and the processes of labor and childbirth. Delivery which takes place too quickly and which is carried out via heavy-handed obstetrical techniques such as artificial hormonal induction, without taking the natural uterine contractions into consideration, is very likely to cause prolapse of the stomach, as well as of other organs (kidneys, bladder, uterus). I have been struck by the high number of gastric prolapses seen in postpartum patients. Fortunately, however, they often resolve themselves.

Uterine retroversion is so common (*Visceral Manipulation*, p. 243) that one forgets that it can affect other visceral articulations. It leaves a space which the greater omentum and small intestine tend to fill up, taking the stomach with them. The perineum (playing the role of an inferior diaphragm) and certain pelvic muscles (e.g., internal obturator) loosen after pregnancy and uterine retroversion. This allows all the organs of the digestive and urogenital systems to move downward.

Abdominal scars, whether of surgical, traumatic or infectious origin, contribute to the destabilization of good visceral disposition.

Predisposing factors listed for hiatal hernia and esophageal reflux (p. 57) may contribute to gastric prolapse as well. Depression and other debilitating illnesses, which may affect postural tone via changes in connective tissues and muscle, are also possible factors.

Some stomachs are congenitally prolapsed. I have seen children in whom the stomach reached the level of the pubis. Often, congenital prolapse is better tolerated than that which is acquired.

I cannot say that skeletal restrictions are causes of prolapses, but their existence does affect gastric mobility. This can be utilized when faced with the failure of manipulating only the stomach itself.

There are also restrictions within the stomach. This organ is like a water-filled balloon inside another water-filled balloon. Air in the stomach rises, forming a superior air pocket. Liquids and solids, on the other hand, collect at the bottom and often lower the level of the pyloric antrum, a phenomenon which can be verified with barium fluoroscopy. The stomach can be filled up without any change in the pressure against its walls. This is because as more is ingested, the walls of the stomach expand, volume increases, and pressure remains constant.

Given a certain density of food (e.g., mashed potato), and bad ingestion habits (fast eating without chewing), internal forces exerted upon the stomach may become excessive. After thousands of meals eaten too quickly, the stomach may become distended more rapidly. I don't believe that this is a major cause of prolapse, but it certainly contributes.

Symptoms

Among the symptoms of gastric prolapse are the following:

- A constant sensation of heaviness in the abdomen, which is worse after meals.
- Deep inspiration increases the discomfort and produces a sense of malaise. I believe that the discomfort is caused in part by the diaphragm pushing down on the stomach, and in part by excessive stimulation of the vagus nerve fibers supplying the cardia. Sometimes, expiration can also be difficult.
- A classic symptom is the need to loosen the belt or some article of clothing while eating.
- Discomfort with straining (coughing, defecation, etc.) is a frequent symptom of prolapse. Stomach pain is often wrongly diagnosed as gastritis (destruction of the stomach cells). I have found through the objective means of endoscopy that irritation and inflammation of the gastric wall can occur without the cellular damage necessary for a diagnosis of gastritis.
- Pyrosis, esophageal reflux and duodenal reflux only accompany serious prolapses.
- Positional discomfort from the arms-up or head-backward positions is common to all prolapses. This is due to the generalized stretching of visceral ligaments and membranes, and probably to stimulation of the vagus and phrenic nerves as well.
- Commonly the patient begins a meal with normal appetite and suddenly is no longer hungry.
- Headache occurring at the end of a large meal.
- When gently shaking the abdomen, one hears a sloshing sound like water being stirred. If this continues long after ingestion of a meal, it signifies incomplete emptying of the stomach.
- The stomach functions at a reduced rate and the patient has the impression of never having finished digesting. This dyspepsia is accompanied by flatulence and frequent belching which are attempts by the body to normalize gastric pressure.
- The patient complains of vertebral and rib pain focused around T6.
- For relief, the patient deliberately induces vomiting in order to empty the stomach and thereby avoid the pulling in the epigastric region due to a full stomach. Vomiting also relieves headaches.
- The patient limits what he eats (because he knows it causes discomfort) and consequently loses weight. Anorexia is not really the appropriate term in this situation as there is no psychiatric component. The word "hyporexia" would be more accurate.
- Radioimaging may reveal a very long stomach in the form of an egg-timer, the pyloric antrum reaching the pubis *(see Illustration 1-6)*.

- The patient assumes a position of forward bending (more pronounced after a meal or at the end of the day) in order to shorten the distance between the gastric fundus and the pyloric antrum. The patient requires a pillow for sleeping.

OTHER DISORDERS

Stomach pains may be of muscular origin (exaggerated stomach contractions and spasms), mucosal origin (burning pain), nervous origin (pain as in the above two types accompanied by nerve pain from the celiac plexus), or a combination.

Functional dyspepsia may be of two types. Hypochlorhydric dyspepsia is characterized by:

- dry mouth with the sensation of an object in the throat
- dysphagia, nausea, headaches, or anorexia
- belching, swelling, or distention
- discomfort or pain before or after breakfast
- good general condition (nervous people have sudden attacks)
- slow and laborious digestion accompanied by a sense of sickness.

Hyperchlorhydric dyspepsia (often confused with gastritis) is characterized by:

- gastric hypertonia
- painful and difficult digestion
- a burning sensation and sour or acid belching after ingestion of sauces, spices, fats, alcohol or tobacco.

The distinction between the two types of dyspepsia is for convenience only. Clinical experience has shown that the hypochlorhydric type can turn, in the space of several days, into the hyperchlorhydric type, and vice versa. In reality, dyspepsia is merely a syndrome which accompanies other illnesses (e.g., neoplasms and appendicitis).

Chronic gastritis is a somewhat abused term, used by some people to refer to a variety of unrelated conditions characterized by stomach pain. In fact, chronic gastritis is a specific disorder characterized by inflammatory infiltration of the submucosal layers of the stomach, and atrophy and dysplasia of the stomach lining. It is a syndrome which may accompany other disorders, including cancer, anemia, polyps, pituitary gland dysfunction, Sjogren's syndrome, etc. It may also be associated with excessive consumption of nitrosamines (in pork or sausages), alcohol, or non-steroid anti-inflammatory drugs, or with duodenal reflux or pernicious anemia. Its symptoms include nausea, rapid loss of appetite on eating, anorexia, vomiting or gastric distention after eating, dyspepsia, bad breath, disagreeable taste in the mouth, and back pain.

Antral gastritis is an antral deformation caused by concentric stenosis, in which the antrum is edematous, hypertrophic and hypomobile.

Duodenal reflux is very frequent in people who drink and smoke. One also finds it in association with restrictions of the pylorus or superior duodenum, ulcers, or surgery on digestive organs. It produces gastritis with atrophied antral mucosa, and may favor development of an ulcer at the acid-alkaline junction at the level of the lesser curvature. I believe that gastric prolapse can produce this problem through liquid aspiration (a type of reflux) caused by an imbalance of intragastric pressures. However, this is merely conjecture based on my clinical observations.

Hypertrophic pyloric stenosis is an uncommon condition in adults, often associated with peptic ulcer near the pylorus. The pylorus is lengthened and stenosed, causing obstruction or retention of the bolus. Sometimes an infiltrating tumor in this area has a similar presentation. In benign conditions, osteopathy is most effective. Another sign is the observation of an abnormal peristalsis which reveals a pyloric obstacle. I occasionally see cases of pyloric stenosis in children. However, I only see mild cases, as more serious ones require surgery. As a diagnostic test, place the child in the supine position, give him a bottle, and observe the abdomen while standing to the right. With pyloric stenosis, you will see the peristaltic waves moving from left to right across the top of the abdomen. Their frequency and amplitude will increase as ingestion continues. At some point, projectile vomiting will occur. Briefly, you will be able to feel the deep pyloric mass, the size of an olive, in the right hypochondrium. The vomiting takes place when stenosis becomes significant. I have treated several cases successfully when the pylorus was not fibrosed and was in spasm, rather than constantly stenosed. With adult stenoses due to ulcers, neoplasms or adhesions, antral dilatation is possible.

Diagnosis

In general listening with a stomach restriction, the patient goes into forward bending, the chin practically resting on the sternum. With restriction of the pyloric and

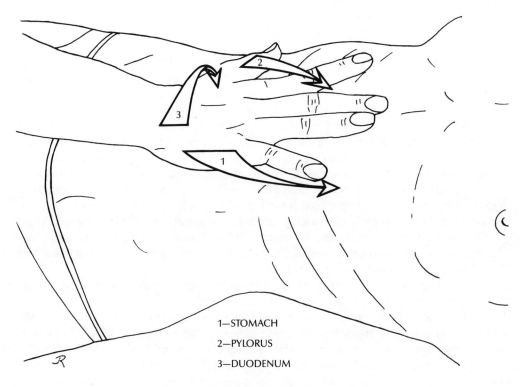

1—STOMACH
2—PYLORUS
3—DUODENUM

Illustration 4-2
Local Differential Diagnosis: Stomach

duodenal regions, this forward bending is accompanied by a slight right sidebending which finishes with a very slight left rotation. General listening gives only approximate results, and must be completed by local differential diagnosis.

LOCAL DIFFERENTIAL DIAGNOSIS

This is performed with the patient in the supine position. Place the palm of your hand underneath the umbilicus, the middle finger on the midline, fingers slightly apart *(Illustration 4-2)*. For the stomach (arrow 1), your entire hand moves upward and to the left, the palm tending to go toward the lower costal margin. For problems of the greater curvature, the hand moves into slight pronation (or for the lesser curvature, into supination), the index finger resting on the lateral edge of the midline. With a prolapse, the palm is drawn toward the pubic region. For the gastroesophageal junction, the middle finger moves toward the xiphoid process and goes past it, the palm moving toward the xiphoidal angle. For the pylorus (arrow 2), the thumb is drawn toward the superior part of the midline below the xiphoid and moves slightly to the left or the right of the midline depending upon the position of the pylorus. It may seem strange to separate the pylorus and the duodenum, but my experience has shown that for ulcers and duodenitis, the hand is drawn to the descending duodenum (arrow 3), and, notably, the sphincter of Oddi (possibly reflecting the role of bile in ulcer formation), in spite of the fact that

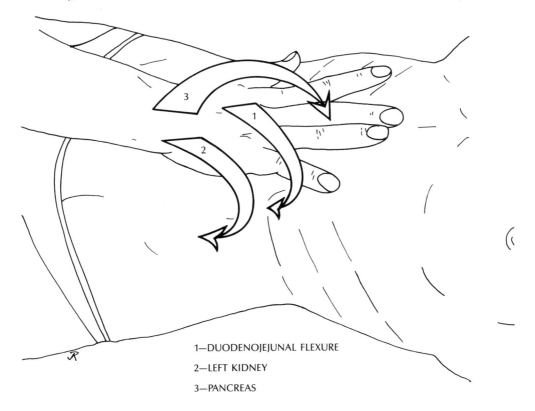

1—DUODENOJEJUNAL FLEXURE

2—LEFT KIDNEY

3—PANCREAS

Illustration 4-3
Local Differential Diagnosis: Duodenojejunal Flexure

more than 95% of duodenal ulcers occur in the superior duodenum. The hand moves to the right, the thumb pushing onto the sphincter of Oddi's projection 2-3 cm above the umbilicus, on a line connecting the umbilicus to the nipple or mid-clavicle. Ulcers, particularly those of the stomach, may attract the hand directly and rotate in a manner similar to the sphincter-like areas.

For restrictions of the duodenojejunal flexure *(Illustration 4-3)*, the hypothenar eminence fixes itself upon the anterior projection (which is symmetrically opposite that of the sphincter of Oddi) and moves deeper until it feels a round mass (arrow 1). For the left kidney (arrow 2), the hand carries out approximately the same movement as described above. However, it remains closer to the umbilicus and goes much deeper posteriorly. Mistakes are commonly made between the duodenojejunal flexure and the left kidney. For the right kidney, the hand is laterally drawn to the right of the umbilicus. It goes past the projection of the sphincter of Oddi, and moves posteriorly while at the same time being subtly drawn toward the thorax if the kidney is in place. For restrictions of the pancreas (arrow 3), the thenar eminence moves toward the projection of the sphincter of Oddi, the hand rotating clockwise until the middle finger makes a 30° angle with the transverse plane perpendicular to the midline at the level of the umbilicus (i.e., a 60° angle with the midline itself).

I cannot review all the situations in which nearby organs confuse or falsify diagnosis. You must learn to recognize "red herring" noises or attractions which have no diagnostic import. Common examples are the stomach's air pocket and the cecum.

DIAGNOSTIC MANIPULATION

If your listening tests suggest a stomach prolapse, confirm this by creating an inhibition point on the lower part of the stomach, pushing it slightly upward. In the case of a prolapse, this inhibition of the stomach will stop the prolapse feeling on listening. The stomach's air pocket is a physiological phenomenon and contributes to maintaining the cardiac notch. Sometimes, for trivial reasons (emotion, eating in a hurry, etc.), it enlarges and consequently interferes with your listening. In this case, with your free hand, gently compress the inferior left costal margin. This is sufficient to remove the irrelevant "noise." For example, let's say your hand is being drawn upward, and you hesitate between implicating the pylorus or the gallbladder. Inhibit the anterior costal projection of the gallbladder; if your hand continues to be drawn upward, you can assume that there is a problem with the pylorus. Alternatively, inhibit the pyloric projection, which should stop the attraction of your hand. Following ulcers, zones of fibrous scar tissue often develop on the lesser omentum, greater omentum, or duodenum. Local listening will allow their detection.

A gastric recoil technique should enable you to differentiate between injury to the attachments vs. the mucosa of the stomach. With the patient in the seated position, place yourself behind him, insert your fingers under the left costal margin, and bring the gastric fundus upward and slightly to the right. At the extreme of this movement, suddenly release the pressure. If the patient feels pain when you compress the stomach, it means that the mucosa is irritated. If the pain occurs during recoil, the attachments (gastrophrenic ligaments, lesser omentum, etc.) are injured. Generally speaking, the patient will be sensitive to both these actions. Make him clearly explain the sensitive point; this way he can indicate to you the zone to be manipulated. Recoil can create sensitivity (and a feeling of nausea) at the level of the gastroesophageal junction because of stretching of the vagus nerves.

As for hiatal hernias (chapter 3), there is an aggravation technique to test for gastric prolapse. Place yourself behind the patient (who is seated and leaning forward) and again insert your fingers under the anterior left costal margin. Bring the fingers slightly upward to collect part of the stomach which you then push downward, toward the umbilicus. With a prolapse, the patient will feel the symptoms he knows only too well, accompanied by a feeling of malaise. For the relief technique, in the same position, gently bring the stomach upward and maintain it there. It is very important to do this gently because these patients often also have hiatus hernias and too vigorous an upward motion could exacerbate that condition. The patient often carries out this relief movement subconsciously.

To manifest a gastric problem, exert compression on the posterior angle of R7 or on the corresponding left costovertebral articulation. For duodenal problems, the compression should be done slightly to the right of the midline. The patient will feel some difficulty in breathing, and an onset or increase of stomach pain. In an alternative backward bending technique, the patient sits with both hands behind the neck. Place yourself behind him and take both elbows, pulling them into passive backward bending. This technique stretches the stomach fibers and irritates points of restriction. In the case of a duodenal problem, the patient will feel discomfort slightly to the right of the midline and will usually try to oppose the movement.

Gastric problems often prevent adequate respiration, mostly of the left hemidiaphragm. In the characteristic relief position of the ulcer sufferer, the patient holds himself in forward bending, the left shoulder downward and slightly forward. If the injury is duodenal, the right shoulder is slightly lowered. Gradually, as mealtime approaches, this position is accentuated. While sleeping, he requires a fairly high pillow (to avoid stretching the stomach fibers), and prefers the right lateral decubitus position with the knees against the chest.

ASSOCIATED SKELETAL RESTRICTIONS

Problems exclusively of the stomach tend to create lower left cervical restrictions, whereas injuries to the pylorus or duodenum give bilateral restrictions, often more evident on the right. In more severe cases, one finds an effect on C7/T1 and R1. The 6th left costovertebral articulation is the epicenter of stomach-related restrictions for this region. Problems of the descending duodenum will be manifested with a similar problem on the right. There are seldom lumbar vertebral restrictions with pure gastric problems, but more often so with duodenal injury.

Left glenohumeral periarthritis is very common, and can be manifested with the glenohumeral articulation test (chapter 1). If the action of slightly bringing the stomach upward improves shoulder movement, you can assume there is gastric reflex injury to the shoulder.

OTHER DIAGNOSTIC CONSIDERATIONS

Minor gastric disorders or inflammation have little effect on the Adson-Wright test, probably because there are relatively few adhesions with surrounding tissues. However, with antropyloric injury resulting from ulcer, the test is generally positive on the left. With injury of the duodenum, it can be positive on the right. You can perform this test in order to confirm the stomach's participation. When there are significant gastric problems, the systolic pressure will be slightly lower on the left.

Other restrictions seen in association with those of the stomach include: left cervical/brachial neuralgia (due to excessive tension of the fasciae which join the stomach to this region, and to irritation of the vagus and phrenic nerves); headache (most often on the left, following the rhythm of gastric peristalsis); lower chest pain (less frequent than with hiatal hernia); and problems of bile transit. The latter begin with extrahepatic biliary problems caused by spasm or restriction of the descending duodenum, whose tension then disturbs flow from the pancreas and gallbladder.

All excretory orifices need good openings for passage of the secreted liquids. At the level of the sphincter of Oddi, nearly two liters per day of secretions from the pancreas and gallbladder should be able to enter the descending duodenum. An imbalanced tension prevents satisfactory opening of the sphincter and circulation cannot take place normally. These digestive fluids then stagnate, irritate their channel, and cause dyspepsia.

Treatment

The stomach is an organ for which many problems can be resolved by appropriate osteopathic manipulation. A stomach which is dysfunctional and in pain loses its mobility and motility; it becomes "frozen" to avoid pain and also because of the fibrosed tissues adhering to it. The posterior part of the stomach, cardia or pylorus may be fixed to nearby structures. The stomach may also suffer from contractions, usually focused around the antropyloric area. I believe that any gastric injury can benefit from osteopathic treatment. The mechanical problems usually involve gastric secretion and general digestive circulation.

DIRECT TECHNIQUE AND RECOIL

Stomach

For local treatment of gastric prolapse, place the patient in the seated position, and apply subcostal pressure. Place the fingers slightly to the left of the midline and direct them posterosuperiorly and very slightly to the right. Relax the pressure and repeat this about ten times. Then leave your fingers in the upper position and bring the patient's entire thorax posterosuperiorly to increase stretching. This is the opposite technique to that for hiatal hernia. I have performed this technique under fluoroscopy, and once obtained superior movement of 15cm for a pyloric antrum which had descended to the level of the pelvis.

Everywhere I go, people ask me, "What is the point of lifting a stomach, and does it always remain in place?" The osteopathic concept of mobility is relevant here. A "lifted" stomach does not, in reality, stay in a superior position, but, on the other hand, never returns to its original position; I have confirmed this many times. More importantly, the stomach regains its mobility and no longer opposes diaphragmatic movement. Through release of the diaphragmatic attachments, the muscle and nerve fibers supplying the stomach are stretched less. A prolapsed stomach means that the whole mass of digestive organs is prolapsed. This phenomenon triggers vasoconstrictive reflexes. The disturbed local circulation (particularly bad venous circulation) causes abdominal pain and digestive problems. Results from visceral manipulation are usually very good in such cases.

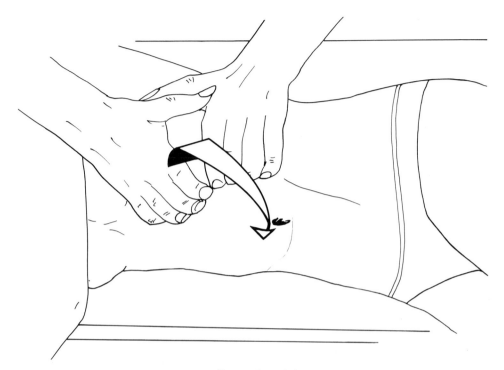

Illustration 4-4
Direct Frontal Technique (Lateral Decubitus Position)

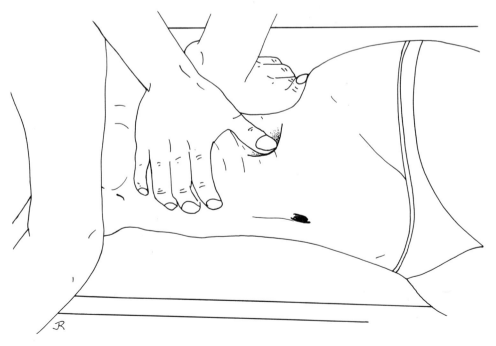

Illustration 4-5
Direct Frontal Technique with Double Lateral Pressure

Recoil can be used when the stomach is unusually sensitive and prolonged pressure is painful. When utilizing recoil, you must treat all parts of the stomach that require work. It may be necessary to shift the focus of your pressure so that you can work on both the left and right parts of the stomach.

I would like you to review the different techniques discussed previously *(Visceral Manipulation,* pages 127-134). Here, I will describe several direct techniques specifically directed to the superior attachments of the stomach, which are very reflexogenic. These techniques consist of mobilizing the attachments on frontal, sagittal and transverse planes. I will first describe two direct frontal techniques.

Have the patient assume the right lateral decubitus position, and stand behind him. Place both hands on the left hemithorax, with the palms below R5 and the fingers over the anterior costal margin. Mobilize the ribs in the direction of the umbilicus, gather

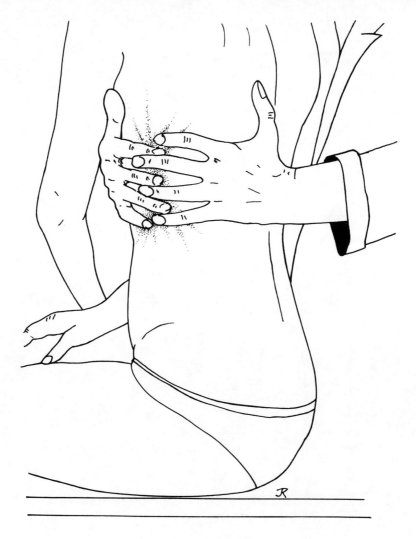

Illustration 4-6
Direct Frontal Technique (Seated Position)

as much of the stomach as possible and put it under the ribs, then stretch it obliquely in a superolateral and posterior direction by bringing your hands back toward you *(Illustrations 4-4 and 4-5)*. Repeat this rhythmically, each time trying to gather more of the stomach, until you feel a release. You then continue the technique by moving your hands farther down the ribs and repeating the movement.

Recoil can be performed when you have carried the ribs as far as possible toward the umbilicus. This is very effective because it enables you to free all the soft tissues on the left which surround the diaphragm, the ribs and the pleura. I often do this two or three times when I begin treating stomach mobility. Alternatively, with the patient in the seated position, sit on his right side and surround his left hemithorax with both hands *(Illustration 4-6)*. Strongly press the ribs inferomedially while supporting the patient against you, and relax suddenly.

A sagittal technique with the patient in the right lateral decubitus position is also possible. Place your right thumb and hand on the posteroinferior part of the left hemithorax. The left hand is in front of the thorax pressing on the 7th through 9th costochondral cartilages. The posterior hand pushes the hemithorax forward while the anterior hand brings it backward, and then vice versa *(Illustration 4-7)*. The gastrophrenic ligaments are thereby engaged. Recoil consists of waiting until both hands have moved as far as possible, and then releasing them simultaneously. This is an efficient and aesthetically pleasing technique as your hands are working separately. When they are synchronized well, there is a perceptible beneficial effect on the body.

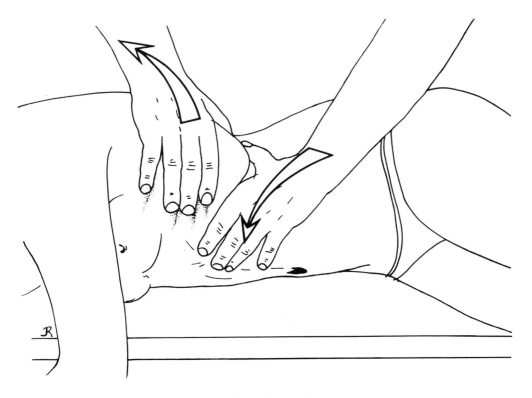

Illustration 4-7
Direct Sagittal Technique (Lateral Decubitus Position)

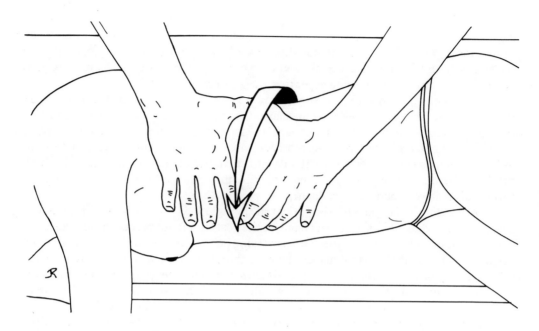

Illustration 4-8
Direct Transverse Technique (Lateral Decubitus Position)

The direct transverse technique is also performed with the patient in the right lateral decubitus position. Place both hands on the anterolateral aspect of the left hemithorax, fingers toward the midline, thumbs toward the back. Both thumbs at the back mobilize the lower ribs, not toward the umbilicus, but toward the xiphoid process (*Illustration 4-8*). This technique has the advantage of mobilizing the posterior gastrophrenic attachments and the sternocostal articulations. Recoil occurs when the hemithorax is at maximal rotation.

Pylorus

One direct technique for the pylorus is performed with the patient supine. When the patient has eaten recently, or is tense, the pylorus is found slightly to the right of the midline (*Illustration 4-9*), four or five fingers' width above the umbilicus. It will generally go into spasm as a result of any type of ulcer, or inflammation of the antrum or duodenum. Pyloric spasm stops gastric mobility and motility, and also brings about spasms of the descending duodenum, which will disrupt transit of digestive fluids from the pancreas and gallbladder. Direct manipulation is performed with a clockwise and counterclockwise compression/rotation combined with transverse pressure. Bring the pylorus toward the left at the end of the clockwise rotation (opening), and toward the right at the end of the counterclockwise movement (closing) in order to increase the stretching effect and help open the pylorus (*Illustration 4-10*). Recoil is performed when you have finished bringing the pylorus transversely to the right or the left as far as you can. It is also used to "awaken" a frozen pylorus. Usually, best results are achieved when your hand moves to the left at the end of the clockwise rotation and to the right at the

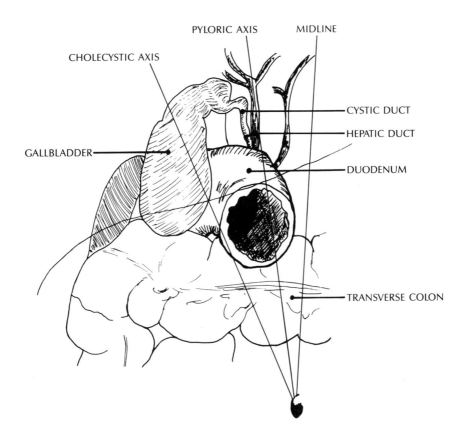

PYLORIC AXIS   MIDLINE

CHOLECYSTIC AXIS

CYSTIC DUCT

HEPATIC DUCT

GALLBLADDER

DUODENUM

TRANSVERSE COLON

Illustration 4-9
Pylorus: Reference Marks

end of the counterclockwise rotation. Recoil must be very quick here in order to have any effect. After two or three repetitions, finish with an induction technique.

Another direct technique for the pylorus has the patient in the right lateral decubitus position. Put both your thumbs in deeply and to the left of the midline, fingers on the medial aspect of the descending duodenum. In order to reach this they have to go past the peritoneum, greater omentum and small intestine. If you are unsure of the location of these organs, begin by looking for the medial part of the ascending colon; against it is the lateral part of the descending duodenum, which serves as a guide for finding the medial part. Your thumbs stretch the pylorus toward the left, while your hands push the duodenal mass to the right. Carry out this technique rhythmically until the spasm ceases and you can move the pylorus without producing pain. This area becomes restricted very deeply and you must be able to explore it at every level. For the recoil technique, let go with the thumbs when they have moved maximally to the right.

The pylorus can be in spasm, fibrosed, even stenosed, the latter condition being manifested by an absolute hardening. The pylorus is a highly reflexogenic zone like the sphincter of Oddi, gallbladder, duodenojejunal flexure, and ileocecal junction. Manipulation of the pylorus stimulates general circulation of the small and large intestine.

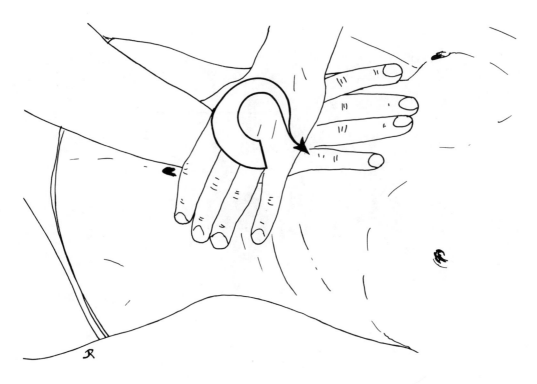

Illustration 4-10
Pylorus: Compression/Rotation

If you have problems getting a reaction, don't hesitate to stimulate the other reflexogenic zones. For example, ileocecal mobilization increases gastric evacuation. Good loosening of the pylorus provokes a characteristic noise from evacuation of liquid (sometimes mistakenly attributed to the gallbladder).

Duodenum

The superior and descending duodenum can be manipulated to stretch the antropyloric region, which is often fixed by adhesions following ulcers. A direct technique with the patient in the seated position again starts with subcostal pressure. Place your fingers slightly to the right of the midline at two fingers' width from the costal margin. Go as deep as possible and bring the fingers back upward against the inferior side of the liver. This presses the bend between the superior and descending duodenum against the liver. Leaving them in this position, pull the patient into backward bending. In this manner you create a vertical longitudinal stretching of the superior and descending duodenum. The lengthening is painful in the case of a restriction. After five or six repetitions, the pain disappears. The recoil technique is performed by quickly letting go after you have pressed the superior and descending duodenum under the liver with your fingers.

I am not yet convinced that it is possible to manipulate the inferior or ascending duodenum in a reproducible manner, and will therefore not try to describe techniques for these areas. However, the duodenojejunal flexure is very important and will be considered with the small intestine in chapter 8.

Sphincter of Oddi

The sphincter of Oddi, another highly reflexogenic zone, is always fixed with injury to the stomach or duodenum. It is found posteroinferiorly inside the descending duodenum, two or three fingers' width above the umbilicus and slightly to the right. It is reached by going across the descending duodenum, and can be transversely manipulated in association with this organ or by direct compression/rotation. For the compression/rotation technique, exert deep pressure with the pisiform on the anterior projection of the sphincter, accompanied by clockwise and counterclockwise rotation, until maximal pressure is reached. At this point, make the pisiform (or the thenar eminence) slide medially and laterally. Finish the technique with recoil and then induction. Again, if loosening takes too long, use the help of the other reflexogenic zones.

INDUCTION

Because the different structures in this area are so closely interrelated (particularly the different parts of the stomach, the duodenum, and the sphincter of Oddi), restriction of one area usually affects the others. This is the situation in which general induction is particularly useful. General induction is usually performed with the patient in the seated position, your left hand on the left costal margin against the gastrophrenic attachments, and your right hand under the liver near the junction of the superior and descending duodenum. Allow the body to move as in an exaggerated form of general listening and it will manipulate itself in concert with your manual pressure.

REMARKS

As a general approach, I like to begin with the sphincter of Oddi, then the pylorus and cardia, because of their reflexogenic properties. Then I manipulate the stomach on its three planes and, finally, the duodenum. As mentioned at the beginning of the chapter, manipulation of the stomach should always be combined with that of the liver (chapter 5). Don't forget the left triangular ligament, which often helps restrict the motion of the stomach.

At the end, listen to the cardia and pylorus. They should both have a clockwise rotation on local listening, i.e., be open. If this is not the case, treat (by induction) the one that goes counterclockwise and check them both again. Repeat this until they both go in a clockwise direction. If this does not happen, you have left something undone that relates to the stomach. Using this technique ensures that the entire stomach is working well· at the end of the treatment.

Recommendations

Always undertake stomach manipulation with care. In the presence of a muscular spasm or irritation of the mucosa, you may increase the irritation, which will set off the patient's defense mechanisms.

The stomach and gallbladder are very closely related because of their shared innervations. Surprisingly, you may find that successful manipulation of the stomach is followed by development of gallbladder problems, or that improvement in the functioning of the gallbladder is accompanied by new stomach problems, and so on. This underscores the importance of treating these structures together.

You must be cautious when treating the stomach, as 30% of ulcers are asymptomatic. Gastric tumors can easily be confused with ulcers. Above all, be wary of cervical and supraclavicular adenopathy, low systolic pressure, short inexplicable syncopes, and enlargement of the spleen or liver, which may indicate more serious pathologies.

ADVICE TO THE PATIENT

Advise patients with stomach problems to avoid clothing and belts which are too tight, and maintaining positions with the arms in the air. In order to counteract stomach acidity, many patients drink large quantities of milk. Initially, this does help relieve the pain. Subsequently, however, the liver and intestines will pay dearly for this short-term improvement. For one thing, the decreased acidity of the stomach will reduce the amount of digestion that occurs there (thereby increasing the load on the small and large intestines). For another, many people have sensitivities or allergies to milk, which puts a burden on the liver.

Sugar taken when fasting (particularly in the late afternoon) is very irritating to the gastric mucosa. Oranges are also badly tolerated in the afternoon. The effects of acidic food and drink depend on the state of acid secretion of the stomach. The more the stomach secretes, the less it accepts these foods, whereas it could need them in the case of hypochlorhydria.

Alcohol and tobacco are not good friends to the stomach. But whose friends are they anyway? I am less dogmatic concerning coffee. It sometimes helps evacuation of the stomach by stimulating smooth muscle activity. However, the long-term harmful effects of caffeine and other components of coffee are undeniable.

Chapter Five:
The Liver

Table of Contents

The Liver

The liver is a large organ with a reputation of being fairly inaccessible. It is protected by the rib cage; its anteroinferior edge does not usually go below the lower costal margin in adults, although in children it may extend 2-3 cm below this margin. Thanks to subcostal techniques *(Visceral Manipulation,* pp. 97-106), it is not difficult to manipulate the liver. Students are always surprised that they are able to put their hands under the liver and lift it up. This organ performs an astonishing variety of functions for the circulatory and digestive systems, and is unfortunately subject to a corresponding variety of restrictions and dysfunctions.

Depending on which medical fad or philosophy you listen to, the liver may be involved in all pathologies or in none. Some so-called healers have actually published statements to the effect that "liver problems" *(mal au foie)* do not exist, and that the disorders commonly attributed to the liver are just part of folklore. However, those of us who work with patients on a daily basis and pay attention to the liver know that it plays a central and crucial role in health, and in the diagnosis and treatment of disease.

Physiology and Anatomy

The liver contacts and is shaped by most of the subdiaphragmatic organs: the hepatic flexure of the colon, right extremity of the transverse colon, right kidney, superior duodenum, gastroesophageal junction, and stomach. It also has close relationships with the peritoneum, pleura, mediastinum, pericardium and the important blood vessels that go through the diaphragm.

Many liver disorders are related to the fact that it is very heavy. Its average weight is probably around 1.5kg, but this can vary considerably depending on age, stage of the digestive cycle, medical history, etc. Actually, because of the "attraction" exerted by the diaphragm *(Visceral Manipulation,* p. 74), the effective weight of the liver is probably around 400g.

The liver is highly vascularized, and may process as much as 1.5 liters of blood per minute. This amount of blood might seem to further exacerbate the problem of heaviness. Actually, the "magnetic" influence of diaphragmatic pressures is reinforced by two circulatory phenomena: a force from the back (the propulsive force of the blood coming from the heart), and another from the front (the aspirational force of the blood leaving the liver as it flows through the vena cava to the heart). These forces of venous circulation contribute to pushing the liver upward against the diaphragm if the heart, blood vessels, etc. are functioning normally.

Circulation within the liver, which normally reinforces diaphragmatic attraction, can become an obstacle if the liver is not flush with the diaphragm, or if it is congested. As previously discussed (chapter 4), pressure immediately below the diaphragm is negative in relation to pressure further down in the abdomen. If the liver is slightly prolapsed (even a few millimeters), heavier because of congestion, or fixed onto a neighboring structure, diaphragmatic attraction cannot play its proper role. The weight of the liver can thus become harmful, increasing its likelihood of separation from the diaphragm.

The forces from the back and the front lose their efficiency when the liver becomes congested. Circulatory stasis affects the sinusoids of the liver and its anastomotic connections to the vena cava (see below), and the patient's entire circulatory system is impaired. You may have noticed that in patients with hepatic dysfunction, the right side is heavy and respiration is impaired, which is not the case with gastric dysfunction.

Proper mechanical functioning of the liver requires the following:

- healthy pleurae and lungs
- supple and tonic diaphragm
- extensible ligamentous attachments
- elasticity of the liver itself
- correct subdiaphragmatic position
- elasticity of hepatic blood vessels
- healthy heart.

With an adult, the simple fact that the practitioner is easily able to palpate the liver in the supine position signifies hepatomegaly or prolapse. Prolapse, also known as a low-lying liver, means that the liver is not enlarged, but merely lower than normal. Usually, on percussion, hepatic dullness will begin at the fourth or fifth intercostal space. With prolapse it may not start until the sixth or even seventh intercostal space. In addition, we have noted that with a prolapse the liver has vertical mobility of 2 cm on palpation in the seated position, whereas vertical mobility in the normal liver is not more than 1 cm. As I have mentioned, the osteopathic concept is more concerned with the mobility of an organ than with its position. Simple detection of a prolapse is not sufficient; is it low and mobile, or low and immobile? The difference is significant.

The liver plays indispensable roles in bile production, formation of plasma proteins, phagocytosis of worn-out blood cells, and metabolism or storage of nutrients and toxins from the digestive system. Innervation of the liver is mostly from the left vagal nerve, celiac plexus, and right phrenic nerve. I will not attempt to describe hepatic physiology in detail here; this is a tremendously complex subject, and my purposes are limited to visceral manipulation and osteopathy. I would, however, like to highlight a few points relevant to discussions of function and pathology presented later in this chapter.

The liver contains roughly 300 billion hepatocytes and has a cumulative secretory pressure of 30 cm H_2O. Biliary secretion is not a simple ultrafiltration, but an active process. Individual cells in the liver last 300 to 500 days and consist of approximately 60% parenchymal hepatocytes, the rest being mostly Kupffer's cells (fixed phagocytic cells found in the sinusoids) and structural framework cells.

The liver is able to accumulate and distribute 1.5 liters of blood per minute, of which 70% comes from the portal vein. The latter is 8 cm long and 1.5 cm wide, and brings to the liver the nutrients absorbed from the small intestine, stomach, and large intestine. The portal system communicates with the inferior vena cava via four groups of anastomoses; esophageal, rectal, umbilical and peritoneal. Balance between flow in the portal vein, hepatic artery, and subhepatic veins, along with vascular resistance, maintains low pressure in the portal system.

There is a complex system of intrahepatic bile capillaries and ducts which merge and leave the liver as the right and left hepatic ducts. These combine to form a common hepatic duct, which in turn unites with the cystic duct from the gallbladder to form the common bile duct emptying into the duodenum. By freeing restrictions of these various ducts, and stretching the surrounding connective tissues, biliary transit is improved. In view of the large quantity of blood circulating through the liver, as well as amount of bile excreted, this restoration of elasticity is clearly important.

Pathology

Factors which can disturb the liver's mechanical functions are of extrahepatic, hepatic and general origin.

There are many possible extrahepatic mechanical factors. A few common examples are scarring or sclerosis of the lungs and pleurae, and hypotonia or fibrosis of the diaphragm. Scars cause adhesion of the liver to adjacent organs after, for example, cholecystectomy or even appendectomy (which increases tension on the ascending colon and thereby destabilizes the lateral part of the liver).

Hepatic factors include the effects of various toxic substances including alcohol and certain drugs and foods. Infections such as viral hepatitis can also cause the liver to lose its natural elasticity. The presence of abnormal fibrous hepatic tissues hinders good circulation and optimal distribution of pressures.

Various general bodily disorders can interfere with hepatic mobility and circulation. For example, hypertrophy of the right ventricle can produce heaviness and blood stagnation in the liver. The coughing associated with chronic bronchitis or asthma, because of the mechanical hammering and enormous pressures it creates, is a source of mechanical liver disorders. Depression, pregnancy, childbirth, sedentary lifestyle, and occupational demands are other commonly implicated factors.

One might expect that an osteopath would see only functional problems. Sometimes, however, we are the first to detect a serious illness, either because it was missed in a medical checkup or because the patient comes to see us first. In this section I will describe some serious liver diseases and specific symptoms which you should learn to recognize as "red flags."

HEPATITIS

There are several types. Type A hepatitis particularly affects children and young adults. Contamination comes from water, milk and seafood, and apparently most people are exposed to this type. Incubation takes 30 days and the disease, if properly treated, usually presents no great danger. It can, however, leave the patient with hepatic hypersensitivity and great fatigue. Type B hepatitis is transmitted via blood (and its derivatives), sperm or saliva. This type is increasing in frequency. It is more serious than type A and leads to a chronic condition in approximately 50% of cases. Some investigators believe that it can favor the development of liver neoplasms. In addition, there is a hepatitis type D (also known as the delta agent), which either coinfects with type B hepatitis or superinfects a chronic carrier of that disease, making the infection more serious and accelerating the destruction of the liver. Finally, some cases of hepatitis do not seem to belong to either of the two common types and are referred to as non-A non-B hepatitis. This form is transmitted in a similar manner to type B and constitutes a very large percentage of the transfusion-related cases of hepatitis in the United States.

Symptoms and Etiology

In hepatitis, the hepatic cells are changed and necrosed, while the reticular network stays intact during the incubation period and the beginning of the acute stage. There is biliary stasis because of bile "corks" and microthrombi in the biliary canaliculi. Prodromes include:

- general feebleness (fatigue, anorexia)
- gastrointestinal problems such as nausea, vomiting, diarrhea
- distortion of the olfactory sense and taste, and aversion to food and tobacco
- joint pain, epigastric discomfort, or a burning sensation in the right hypochondrium.

Type A hepatitis may also be characterized by 39-40°C fever, flu-like symptoms, coughing, coryza, pharyngitis, muscle soreness, photophobia, dark urine (from bilirubin), discolored stools, severe itching, or enlargement and sensitivity of the liver.

In any type of hepatitis, a jaundiced or icteric phase can occur after 6 weeks. In this phase, there is a 3-5kg weight loss, the stools get darker, acne can develop during the second week, and the liver is enlarged and painful (this diminishes in 15 days). In 20% of cases one also finds posterior cervical adenopathy and splenomegaly.

When there is no jaundice (anicteric hepatitis), the disease may be characterized by fever, intestinal transit problems, gastroenteritis, respiratory infections (in children), hepatomegaly, hepatic pain on palpation, and anorexia. Unfortunately, any or all of these symptoms may be absent. Nonicteric hepatitis may be confused with influenza, gastroenteritis, or mononucleosis (which causes serious and painful adenopathy, pharyngitis and splenomegaly).

In *persistent chronic hepatitis*, which comprises about 10% of cases, hepatomegaly can last several years. The function of the liver is only intermittently normal. With biopsy one sees mononuclear infiltration, slight portal fibrosis, and degeneration of the hepatocytes.

In *drug-induced hepatitis*, the liver is hypersensitive to certain chemicals or drugs. Immunological responses are apparently involved in these cases, which are often characterized by joint pain, intense itching, and fever. The liver is often sensitive to testosterone and estrogen, and it has been suggested that its excretory functions are reduced by oral contraceptives. Barbiturates are known for their hepatic toxicity, but this results more from the interaction of the medicine and the person, rather than the medicine itself (unless it is taken in enormous doses). For example, some people are able to tolerate large doses of phenobarbital while others become ill from a very small amount. Hepatitis-like illnesses may also be caused by other viruses (Epstein-Barr, cytomegalovirus, etc.), alcohol, hypotension or biliary tract disorders.

Active chronic hepatitis follows or results from acute hepatitis, drug intoxication or disturbance of immune function. This is a progressive, inflammatory, destructive liver disease, affecting mostly adolescents and young women, which leads to fibrosis, necrosis, and finally cirrhosis. Its early symptoms (fatigue, acne) are unremarkable, but these are followed by jaundice, fever, diarrhea, amenorrhea, abdominal and joint pain, hepatomegaly, splenomegaly and spider angiomas. Pain is felt in the major joints, and this is often the symptom leading the patient to seek treatment.

CIRRHOSIS

Cirrhosis can result from a variety of long-term pathologies affecting the liver, e.g., hepatitis, biliary cirrhosis, Wilson's disease (hepatolenticular degeneration), chronic congestive heart failure, or schistosomiasis. Histological characteristics of cirrhosis include reduction in hepatocyte number, destruction and fibrosis of the reticular support system, and anomalies of the vascular layer. General clinical symptoms include jaundice, edema or ascites, disorders of coagulation, portal hypertension with esophageal and gastric varicose veins, splenomegaly, encephalopathy and cachexia.

Alcoholic

Alcoholic cirrhosis (also known as Laënnec's cirrhosis) is the common type in the industrialized world. A result of chronic and excessive alcohol consumption, it causes fine and diffuse sclerosis of the liver, along with decreasing density, progressive loss of hepatocytes, and fatty infiltration. Several small areas of healthy or regenerated parenchyma can persist and form nodules. Clinical symptoms may include some (but not necessarily all) of the following: general fatigue, anorexia, weight loss, hepatomegaly and splenomegaly, distended abdomen, edema at the ankles, muscular atrophy, hair loss, pigmented skin, testicular atrophy, gynecomastia, distention of the parotid and lacrimal glands, clubbing with round nails, palmar erythrosis, Dupuytren's contracture, jaundice, spider angiomas, purpura, and hepatic encephalopathy with confusion.

Other cirrhoses do exist, including cardiac cirrhosis, metabolic cirrhosis, and forms that develop after infectious diseases such as brucellosis or schistosomiasis. However, I am not trying here to replace a textbook of internal medicine. I will describe one additional type which is relatively frequent.

Biliary

Biliary cirrhosis results from disruption of bile excretion, with histological evidence of hepatocyte destruction occurring around the extrahepatic bile ducts. It is often asymptomatic. Approximately 90% of symptomatic cases occur in women between the ages of 35 and 60. We can differentiate primary and secondary biliary cirrhosis. The primary form involves chronic hepatic cholestasia (stoppage of bile excretion), apparently under the partial influence of female hormones. The secondary form involves obstruction of the principal bile ducts (by gallstones, tumor, postoperative stricture, etc.).

Obstruction of the extrahepatic bile ducts in biliary cirrhosis causes a number of secondary effects, including centrolobular biliary stasis, degeneration or necrosis of hepatocytes, proliferation and dilatation of ducts and ductules, and inflammation of the bile ducts with infiltrations. Cholesterol deposition increases, and the portal fissure dilates because of edema and becomes fibrosed. Bile can collect and form biliary lakes. The liver changes color to yellow and green and, as the disease progresses, becomes nodular.

Clinical symptoms of biliary cirrhosis may include:

- hepatomegaly, progressive and prolonged jaundice
- dark urine, intense itching, diarrhea or steatorrhea
- purpura, periorbital xanthelasma, or cutaneous xanthomas
- malabsorption of lipid-soluble vitamins, leading to night blindness (vitamin A), dermatitis (vitamin E and/or essential fatty acids), bone pain from osteomalacia (vitamin D), or easy bruising (vitamin K).

OTHER DISORDERS

Portal Hypertension

This condition usually results from cirrhosis, or mechanical obstruction of the portal vein due to thrombosis or tumor proliferation. It leads to development of a collateral venous circulation, which in turn may cause hemorrhoids, or varicose veins of the gastroesophageal region, retroperitoneal space, ligamentum teres (round ligament of the liver), or periumbilical region (in the latter case producing a venous rosette [caput medusae] around the umbilicus.

Major complications of portal hypertension include (1) rupture of the varicose veins in the gastric fundus and lower esophagus, with massive hematemesis or melena; and (2) hepatic encephalopathy.

Once, in a pulmonary ward, I witnessed a case of ruptured esophageal varicose veins due to coughing. The patient lost approximately one liter of blood which was projected as far as the ceiling, due to combined forces of coughing and pressure in the varicose veins. Such dramatic cases are rare; more common are small functional portal hypertensions.

The mechanism of hepatic encephalopathy is not well understood. However, since ammoniemia (excessive concentration of ammonia in the blood) is sometimes associated with encephalopathy, it is believed that ammonia plays an important part. With ammoniemia, nitrated substances (primarily protein) absorbed in the intestine are not metabolized by the liver before being sent back into general circulation, and the patient must be told to severely limit protein ingestion.

Lipid Infiltration

The mild hepatomegaly observed in this condition is due to infiltration of hepatocytes by fats, triglycerides, phospholipids, and cholesterol. This fatty degeneration can lead to abdominal pain, dyspepsia, or anorexia. The liver is large and firm on palpation. Lipid infiltration may result from alcoholism, diabetes, obesity, ulcerative colitis, pancreatitis, cardiac insufficiency, or hepatotoxic agents such as DDT, phosphorus, varnish, and paint.

Hepatoma

Hepatomas (liver tumors) may be primary or secondary. Technically, hepatomas develop from the hepatocytes, and cholangiomas from the bile ducts, but these two types of carcinoma are often found together. Hepatoma is 2-4 times more common in men than in women. The incidence of this disease is fairly low in Europe and America, but quite high in Africa and Asia. About 70% of patients with hepatoma also have cirrhosis. Symptoms of hepatoma include moderate epigastric and right hypochondrial pain, friction rubs or bruit over the liver, and blood-tinged ascites. Jaundice is an uncommon finding.

Secondary tumors are twenty times more common than primary ones. These metastatic deposits from primary tumors located elsewhere tend to appear in the liver due to its processing functions and its dual blood supply (i.e., hepatic artery and portal vein). All types of cancer (except primary cerebral tumors) can cause metastases to the liver. Symptoms may include:

- those of the original tumor
- fatigue, weight loss, fever, sweating, anorexia
- symptoms of hepatic injury, e.g., hepatomegaly, splenomegaly, a hard, painful liver, or hepatic friction rubs.

ASSOCIATED FACTORS

In this section, I will briefly discuss some associated factors of clinical interest in hepatic disorders.

I must emphasize that intensity of pain does not necessarily indicate the seriousness of an illness. With hepatoma, for example, liver pain is moderate at the beginning and may be mild when the patient comes for consultation.

Many people develop hepatitis without being aware of it. They first learn about it during a general physical examination or after debilitating functional problems such as general fatigue, depression, or serious hypotonia. Hepatitis remains in some ways a poorly-understood disease, particularly in regard to its relationship with the mind. For example, one can have a stomach disease and maintain a high level of mental and psychological concentration; this is not true with hepatitis, but the reason is unknown. Extremely often in osteopathy, we find severe restrictions (actual fixations) of the liver. It is my belief that hepatitis and/or nervous breakdown is often responsible for this phenomenon.

Oral Contraceptives

In the specialized medical literature, one often reads about the damage which oral contraceptives can cause to the liver. They can lead to hepatic cholestasia with or without symptoms such as intense itching, jaundice, and dark urine. Patients who experience recurring idiopathic jaundice or severe itching during pregnancy have increased risk of developing hepatotoxicity due to oral contraception. During pregnancy, nausea or vomiting is due, among other causes, to high levels of estrogen which diminish the excretory capacity of the liver.

Diet

Diet plays a primary role in hepatic metabolism. It is common knowledge that many alcoholics manage to hide their dependence from even their immediate family and close friends. Women use make-up to hide the external ravages of alcoholism. They, more often than male alcoholics, develop joint pains which are difficult to treat. With patients of either sex who have a sensitive liver, the muscular and ligamentary systems will generally benefit from carefully restricted intake of proteins and fats. This recommendation is based on my observation that people who avoid meat and cheese have, in general, fewer hepatic problems, as well as fewer spinal problems. Perhaps this is because diet plays a large part in determining the level of uric acid in the body. A high level of uric acid is harmful to both the liver and the joints.

Joint Pain

This symptom is fairly common with hepatic injury and is one of many examples of the connection between visceral and musculoskeletal disorders. I remember one patient who suffered from right knee pain which I was unable at first to treat successfully. The knee pain spontaneously resolved for three years, and then returned with increased severity. This patient was suffering from a relapse of type B hepatitis, which she had not revealed at first. The relapse, along with an ordinary small twisting movement of the knee, had brought back the knee pain. Osteopathic treatment helped temporarily, but when she stopped drinking alcohol the knee pain disappeared for good within two months. I would also like to mention right glenohumeral periarthritis which, apart from rare direct trauma, is often the reflection of a hepatobiliary malfunction, discussed below.

The liver is an important part of the circulatory system, and I believe that external manipulation of the liver affects its circulation. The circulatory system responds to stimulation of mechanoreceptors and pressure receptors via the nervous system, and to direct stretching of perivascular tissues (which often lose their elasticity when injured).

With serious liver problems there is the risk of a hepatic encephalopathy, which can bring about serious behavioral problems. Beside this serious pathology, there are milder mental problems which can be induced by cholestasia. The hepatic patient is often depressed and tires easily, not necessarily in proportion to the seriousness of the disease. Successful treatment of the liver can relieve this type of depression. Oriental medicine postulates a connection between the liver and the mind. Could this connection be primarily due to ammoniemia?

Dysfunction of the liver has a rapid effect on the skin; itching, xanthoma, xanthelasma, and acne are frequent manifestations. It is therefore important to observe the patient's skin while performing a physical examination. In this respect, it is helpful to have the patient undress as much as possible.

Diagnosis

GENERAL

In diagnosis of hepatic dysfunctions, observation is very important. With liver restrictions, the patient carries himself forward bent and in right sidebending in order to relax the perihepatic membranous tensions. There are other signs of functional problems which do not threaten the life of the patient, but which are enough to prevent a decent quality of life. The most important of these symptoms are:

- hormonal dependence of female digestion
- nightly hyperthermia (at around 2 A.M. for the liver and 4 A.M. for the gall-bladder) which is often accompanied by discomfort in the right lateral decubitus position
- sensation of heaviness in the hypochondrium, with chest wall pain, on the right side
- photophobia experienced one or two hours after mealtimes (when the liver is working the hardest)
- facial swelling and flushing, primarily on the right, during the same time period
- bilateral headache often accompanied by neck pain
- chronic sinusitis, sensitive or irritated sinuses, abnormally sharp sense of smell
- hypersensitivity of the eyeball, increased intraocular pressure
- hypersensitivity of the scalp
- minor disequilibrium and difficulty changing position
- vertigo which is more intense at certain times of the day (on awakening, at the end of the afternoon, and at bedtime)
- gritty tongue, acetonic breath
- oily skin, greasy hair and hair loss
- sleep which leaves one feeling unrested, difficulty in awakening, morning tired-ness which continues during the day.

There are some similarities to disorders of the stomach, particularly in relation to sleep and fatigue. However, the stomach seems to affect the more superficial energy. For example, there may be morning tiredness with stomach disorders, but it will dissipate as the day progresses.

Initial Exam

During the initial exam, the patient's answers to your questions are very important. Gastroenterologists believe that most people suffer, at some time, from type A hepatitis. In addition, types B, D and non-A non-B hepatitis (see above) are becoming more common due to their association with drug use and sexually-transmitted diseases. The effect on the liver of any of these forms of hepatitis is permanent.

In hepatic cases, questioning should address each of these factors: (1) Personal, familial or hereditary hepatic antecedents. (2) Time spent in the third world (i.e., risk of amebiasis, malaria or other parasitic diseases). However, be aware that parasites can be contracted in industrialized as well as third world countries. Parasitic disease should be suspected in a patient who frequently scratches the nose, anus and eyes. (3) Tendency toward hemorrhaging (nasal, ecchymotic or hemorrhoidal). (4) Possible sources of toxicity (such as chemicals, drugs or alcohol). Be particularly alert for alcoholic addiction which the patient attempts to conceal. Alcoholism touches all levels of society and is prevalent in both men and women. (5) Alimentary and sexual habits.

In my opinion, there is little point in treating people who poison themselves daily (with alcohol, cigarettes, drugs or junk food), as these people are not willing to do the work it takes to help themselves. You should have no illusions about the efficacy of your treatments on such people; usually the beneficial effects will last only a few days. It is similarly difficult to treat people with active sexually-transmitted diseases. These diseases affect the liver and when you try, through manipulation, to induce self-healing it cannot respond effectively because all its energy is being used against the consequences of the disease. I believe that in these cases it is better for the patient to undergo appropriate drug therapy before beginning manipulative treatment. Often people have sexually-transmitted diseases without knowing it (most commonly *Chlamydia*). If you are working on a hepatic case and are disappointed by the results, ask the patient to undergo laboratory examination to determine whether or not he has a sexually-transmitted disease.

Evaluation of Symptoms

On *percussion and palpation*, anterior hepatic dullness can stretch from the fifth intercostal space to the inferior costal margin. Percussion enables one to evaluate positioning, atrophy, hepatomegaly, and the liver's sensitivity to touch. With the stethoscope, hearing friction rubs indicates inflammation and microadhesions of the peritoneal surfaces. These can also be manifested by the hepatic relief movement, which produces a characteristic crackling sound. In the phenomenon known as Murphy's sign, moderate pressure on the gallbladder surface projection produces pain which is also awakened by deep inhalation. However, a subcostal palpation described below is more precise. For the test of hepatojugular reflux, exert a slight pressure on the liver and maintain it for approximately thirty seconds. If swelling of the jugular veins appears, and then disappears when the pressure is lessened, you should think about right ventricular insufficiency. Take note of the abdominal venous dilatations with corresponding collateral circulation from compression of the inferior vena cava leading to engorgement of the portal vein. Cases of serious right cardiac insufficiency will also cause congestion and distortion of the liver.

Some general *digestive problems* such as anorexia, slow and laborious digestion, nausea, vomiting, abdominal distention, and gritty tongue are not very specific for liver disorders. More distinctive symptoms include:

- morning vomiting of a thick, viscous liquid (common with alcohol toxicity), bitter regurgitations
- alimentary intolerance which often leads to pain after ingestion of fatty foods, eggs or chocolate
- urgent diarrhea after eating (alternating diarrhea and constipation are often found with bad biliary evacuation or gallstones)
- persistent discoloration of stools (grayish, ash or putty-colored), which signifies inadequate biliary excretion, or an absence of stercobilin in the stools. This symptom must be differentiated from the yellowish fatty stools associated with pancreatic insufficiencies, and the frothy yellowish stools from problems of the colon.

Dull pain is not very precisely localized and is therefore relatively difficult to analyze. It can be referred to the vertebral column, ribs, shoulders, or abdomen, and has several possible causes. If the pain is provoked by stress or consumption of foods such as eggs, cream, pork meat, fats, fried foods, or white wine, consider infection of the gallbladder, or gallstones. Acute infection of the bile ducts is manifested by sharp, pulsating pain accompanied by an increase of temperature (these signs can also accompany acute hepatitis). Hepatomegaly is revealed by an unpleasant feeling of weight and painful discomfort on the right side, radiating to the shoulders. Hepatic congestion, accompanied by a sense of oppression, cyanosis and labored breathing with effort are often of cardiac origin. Passive congestion with liquid retention is of cardiac origin, whereas active inflammatory congestion often follows hepatitis.

Palpation

Hepatic manipulation is often carried out in the seated position using subhepatic manual pressure. It is important that you recognize the various organs in relation to the inferior side of the liver, and that you know how to evaluate its consistency.

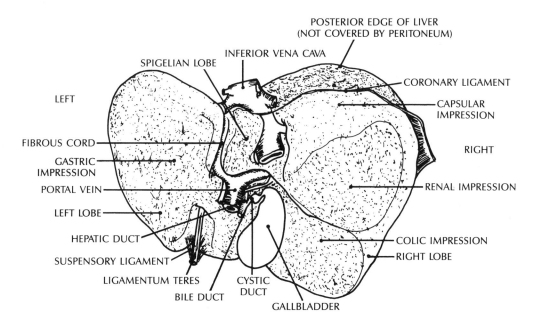

POSTERIOR

Illustration 5-1
Liver: Inferior Surface

From right to left at the front are found: the impressions of the ascending colon, the gallbladder, the quadrate lobe, and the grooves of the ligamentum teres and the stomach. At the back: the right kidney, spigelian lobe, inferior vena cava and stomach *(Illustration 5-1)*. It is very difficult to separate these elements. After many years of practice I still have problems. The gallbladder and right kidney are often sensitive to palpation.

The liver mass is normally fairly smooth. Hepatic palpation is normally painless except for the gallbladder and, posteriorly, the right kidney. It is essential that you know the different pathological signs that can be felt by hepatic palpation *(Dousset, 1964)*:

- A moderate but discrete hepatomegaly, painless, with multiple small, closely spaced protrusions ("hobnail liver") indicates cirrhosis, often of alcoholic origin
- Hardness with "chestnut" protrusions, less numerous than in the preceding case ("uneven liver"), is characteristic of nodular neoplastic infiltrations
- A liver covered with grooves ("tied-up liver") indicates a sclerotic framework typical of syphilis
- The presence of 3-4 regular, round prominences which seem to shake on palpation indicates a hydatid cyst
- One or more rounded, mobile prominences, very painful on palpation and accompanied by fever and alteration of general condition, means a liver abscess
- A massive, hardened hepatomegaly which does not move with inhalation could be due to a primary hepatoma.

To conclude, if the liver does not have normal consistency and smoothness, or if it is painful outside the vesicular and renal zones, discuss with the patient the possible causes, and make sure that he undergoes appropriate diagnostic testing to rule out cancer and other serious pathologies.

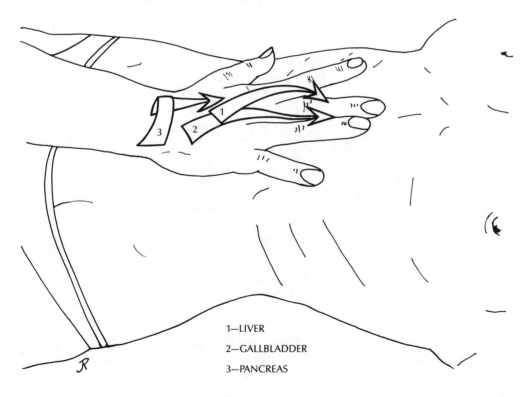

1—LIVER
2—GALLBLADDER
3—PANCREAS

Illustration 5-2
Local Differential Diagnosis: Liver

OSTEOPATHIC

On general listening, the patient (in the seated position) carries out a right side-bending accompanied by a very slight left rotation around an axis which goes through R9-10 on the right. This is also the most comfortable position for hepatitis sufferers.

Differential Diagnosis

At the beginning of local differential diagnosis, the palm of the hand is applied above the umbilicus, the middle finger resting on the midline, the fingers slightly apart (*Illustration 5-2*). The palm is drawn toward the right hypochondrium, rotates clockwise and moves superiorly. The thenar eminence moves toward the right costal margin. For the *gallbladder*, the palm only carries out very slight clockwise rotation, while the index finger and thenar eminence are placed on the midclavicular-umbilical line and then deeply under the costal margin. For the *sphincter of Oddi and pancreatic head*, the hand pronates slightly so that the thenar eminence moves in deeply on the midclavicular-umbilical line, 3cm above the umbilicus, and is directed at a 30° angle from the transverse plane. At the end of the movement, the hand is only resting on the thenar eminence. For the *pylorus*, the hand moves toward the xiphoid process, moving slightly to the left or the right depending on the position of the pylorus. As a general rule, the pylorus is found 6-7cm above the umbilicus, to the left or right of the midline depending on whether the stomach is (respectively) empty or full. However, its position is highly variable (see chapter 4).

For differential diagnosis of the *right kidney*, the thenar eminence moves toward the right (*Illustration 5-3*). However, it does not move upward in a subcostal direction. At the end of the movement it is pulled deeply into the abdomen, 2-3cm to the right of the umbilicus. For the *ascending colon*, the hand, with a significant clockwise rotation, moves toward the ascending colon and then into the abdomen. For the *hepatic flexure*, the hand rotates clockwise and moves toward the most lateral part of R10-11.

Adson-Wright Test

With hepatic dysfunction, this test is often positive, the pulse diminishing or disappearing on the right side, even without left rotation of the head. This positive result may be caused by tension of the hepatic fasciae. If the simple act of lifting the liver improves circulation of the right upper limb, you should look for problems of the liver, kidneys, and hepatic flexure. Remember that these organs are suspended from the liver. If participation of the liver is confirmed, systolic pressure on the right should be restored following successful treatment. In the case of a third degree renal prolapse (a kidney which has lost its attachment to the liver), the hepatic lifting technique no longer affects it, and there will be no effect on the Adson-Wright test.

DIAGNOSTIC MANIPULATION

The area between the inferior edge of the right ribs and the umbilicus is certainly one of the most complex to investigate and often requires inhibition techniques in order to render diagnosis precise. I shall only describe some sample techniques, leaving it to the practitioner to apply these principles to the organs which are not mentioned.

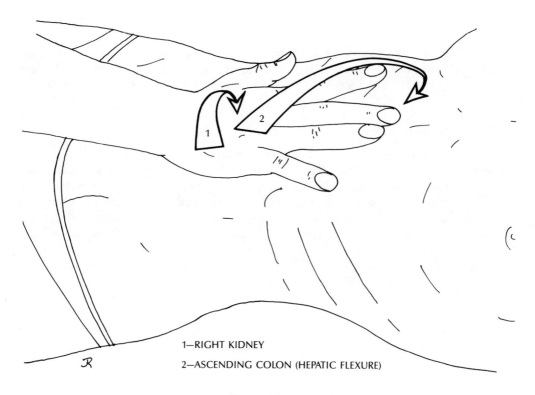

1—RIGHT KIDNEY
2—ASCENDING COLON (HEPATIC FLEXURE)

Illustration 5-3
Local Differential Diagnosis: Right Kidney

Inhibition

As one example, let's say your hand is drawn toward the liver without your knowing whether the liver, gallbladder, or hepatic flexure of the colon is involved. With the other hand, look for the motility of the liver and fix it in its neutral position halfway between inspir and expir. If your hand is no longer drawn toward the liver, this could be the source of the problem. Inhibition of the motility in this manner is the most precise method of testing whether a certain organ is or is not the source of a problem.

Now, suppose that inhibiting the liver has no effect on the movement of the hand. The problem then involves either the gallbladder or the hepatic flexure. Inhibit the surface projection of the gallbladder found on the midclavicular-umbilical line at its costal intersection. If the palm still moves upward and to the right, you can conclude that there is a problem of the hepatic flexure.

The inhibition technique can seem either simple or complex depending on the ability of your hand. It requires long apprenticeship and, once mastered, enables you to be very precise. If others are unconvinced, this precision can be objectively demonstrated using imaging techniques such as fluoroscopy, ultrasound or scanning.

Aggravation/Relief

With hepatic injury, the liver is often sensitive and congested. The simple act of limiting its mobility can aid diagnosis. Suppose that you are hesitating between diagnosing a problem of the liver vs. the pancreas. One technique that will help you determine whether the liver is involved is to press with one hand on the posterior angles of R7-9 on the right *(Illustration 5-4)*. If there is no problem with the liver, there will be no discomfort. If there is a liver problem, this pressure will be uncomfortable and even painful. Also, in patients with liver problems, as you follow the slight amount of motion that is there, respiration will become more difficult, and the sense of discomfort in the hepatic region will increase. In severe cases, the simple costal pressure causes the patient to hold his breath.

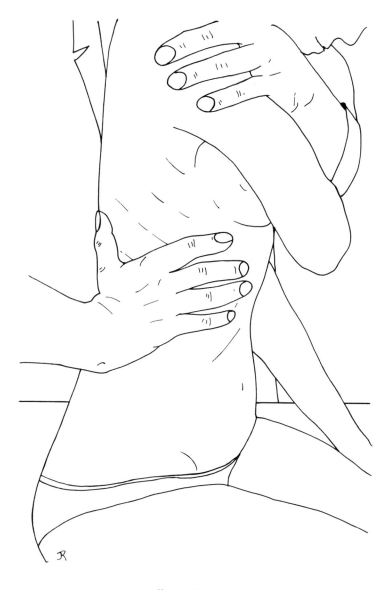

Illustration 5-4
Costal Pressure Technique

Relief maneuvers are less easily performed than those for the stomach. You can accompany the liver during exhalation and then maintain it. If this relieves hepatic discomfort, you can assume that the liver is the cause. But this would be to ignore all the organs suspended from the liver. I prefer to lift the liver, in conjunction with initial pressure on the posterior and lateral angles of the ribs. With hepatic problems, R7-9 are sensitive to this type of pressure. If the sensitivity disappears as you lift the liver, this supports the idea of hepatic involvement.

Lift

Of all the viscera, the liver is certainly the easiest to move completely. The liver lift is performed with the patient in the seated position and the practitioner behind him. Utilizing the direct subcostal approach, put your fingers below the liver and lift it up (see also *Visceral Manipulation*, pp. 92-3). Immediate provocation of pain signifies that the actual hepatic tissue is affected. If pain is felt when the liver is passively returning to its original position, a problem of its ligamentary attachments is indicated.

With serious problems of the liver (such as hepatitis), Glisson's capsule, the liver and its attachments all become sensitive. The liver lift is particularly useful in patients with chronic hepatic disorders, in whom the liver is heavier than normal and Glisson's capsule less supple; i.e., the liver itself is sensitive and so are its attachments (as they are strained by the increased weight).

ASSOCIATED SKELETAL RESTRICTIONS

Restrictions of *thoracic vertebrae and ribs* are well-known and fairly characteristic with hepatic injury; they typically involve T7-T10 and R7-10. Costovertebral mobility tests are disturbed and compression of the spinal and transverse vertebral processes, or the posterior angles of the ribs, creates liver sensitivity. A primary costothoracic restriction does not permit any movement during mobility tests, whereas a secondary restriction of hepatic origin may permit limited movement. This relationship between the ribs and the liver does not only go in one direction; a direct fall on the ribs can result in lifelong hepatic problems.

Liver problems often result in right or bilateral cervical vertebral restrictions (initially at the level of C4-5), while gallbladder problems usually lead to problems on the left. This ipsilateral restriction can be explained both by the interplay of the right cervical/pleural fasciae and the irritation of the vagus and right phrenic nerves. The more the liver is affected, the more the lower cervical and first thoracic vertebrae (and first rib) are restricted.

Glenohumeral periarthritis is found mostly on the right when related to liver dysfunction. Glenohumeral periarthritis of traumatic origin is less common than that attributable to an organ. When there is shoulder pain secondary to liver problems, there is usually also simultaneous pain around C4-5.

The liver also affects the *cranium and face*. Many right-sided cranial base restrictions are secondary to those of the liver. In addition, the right frontal/nasal articulation is a trigger point for the liver.

The liver attaches itself to the diaphragm and pleura, and the latter to the cervical column and ribs. Any abnormal tension of the liver can be transmitted by this system of attachments and directly irritate the cervical/brachial plexuses and associated fasciae.

To obtain confirmation of hepatic involvement, perform the glenohumeral articulation test (see chapter 1) while lifting the liver. If the shoulder's mobility is noticeably improved by the lifting, you may conclude that there is a problem of the hepatic fasciae. If inhibition of the hepatic region improves the shoulder's mobility, this indicates a problem of the liver itself. If there is no improvement at the shoulder with either of these techniques, the problem is most likely with some other organ, or with the shoulder itself.

People with hepatic problems often breathe primarily with their left hemi-diaphragm. In order to alleviate the discomfort and decrease the amount of work necessary for breathing, the diaphragm seems to respond by relaxing the right phrenohepatic attachments. You can use this phenomenon to evaluate the results of your treatments. At the end of the session, the left and right parts of the thorax should move together smoothly, indicating harmonious diaphragmatic respiration.

Although *sciatica* of purely discal origin does exist (see chapter 1), this disorder is more commonly of visceral origin. In regard to the liver, it is important to separate left vs. right sciaticas. With left sciatica, a significant collateral venous circulation develops as a result of portal hypertension. At the rectosigmoid level, the hemorrhoidal veins are dilated, causing inflammation and congestion of the sacral region. My experience indicates that the epidural veins which depend on the azygous system are also congested and dilated, to such an extent that a left sciatica of venous hepatic origin can occur. These forms of sciatica are very acute and unresponsive to medical treatment or physical therapy. They are not to be manipulated at the lumbosacral region as this can increase the irritation of the local tissues. For left sciatica, perform a Lasègue test with an inhibition point at the sigmoid and then the liver. This is the most efficient technique and can indicate the first region to be manipulated.

With right sciatica, hepatic participation may result from disturbance of the hepatic fasciae, right kidney, ascending colon, psoas or lower limbs. This symptom is often found with fibrosis of the liver and/or its attachments. The Lasègue test is carried out with direct inhibition of the liver and, when positive, the gain should be considerable. My experience, in general, is that right-sided sciaticas are relatively easier to treat than those on the left.

Restrictions of the left lower limb correspond more to problems of the hepatic vein and inferior vena cava. They are rarely fascial or mechanical joint restrictions, whereas right restrictions often are. The most common mechanical restrictions in my experience have involved the lateral part of the right lower limb, including the proximal and distal tibiofibular articulations, cuboid, and fifth metatarsal.

Treatment

The osteopathic approach requires looking at each case on an individual basis. It does not allow one to make up a list of simple rules on the order of "hepatitis = such and such a technique" and "cirrhosis = another technique," etc. I treat the liver whenever the hepatic and perihepatic tissues lose their natural elasticity.

Manipulation of the liver clearly has an effect on its metabolism, and on its role in the digestive, endocrine and immune systems. I have achieved good clinical results with my treatments but, unfortunately, have not yet been able to obtain formal quantitative proof of these effects (e.g., improvement in standard liver function tests after manipulation).

Where there are definite signs of portal hypertension, be very careful with direct manipulation. The vessels and hepatic tissues will be quite fragile. A fever accompanying the classical hepatic symptoms can signify viral hepatitis. I am not certain whether manipulation is advisable in an evolving hepatitis; it is certainly useful in the sequela period. I also recommend great caution in the presence of weight loss, anorexia, mild fevers, cervical adenopathy, hepatomegaly and splenomegaly, hepatic rubs, or irregular and painful subhepatic palpation.

Local treatment consists essentially of stretching and stimulating the liver attachments and liberating the bile ducts. For the liver attachments which are deep and subcostal, work via the ribs and the liver itself. For example, to stretch the right triangular ligament, lift the liver by its right extremity and let it return to its original position. The stretching of the ligament will occur during the return phase. Be sure to work on all three planes (frontal, sagittal and transverse) when treating this ligament.

In the remainder of this section I will describe some new techniques, assuming (as I have throughout this book) that the reader is familiar with those presented in *Visceral Manipulation*.

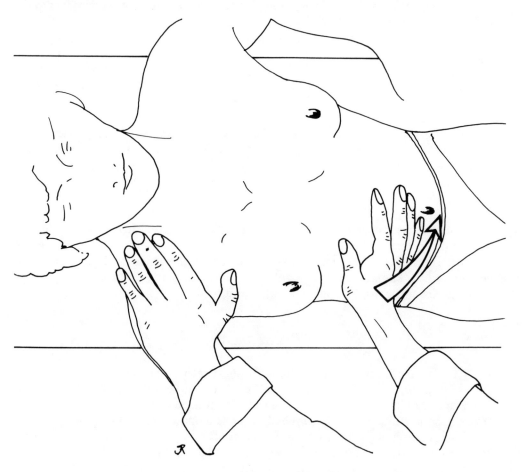

Illustration 5-5
Indirect Manipulation of the Liver (Frontal Plane)

RECOIL

An effective recoil technique, with the patient in the seated position, can be carried out while lifting the liver. Stand behind the patient, hands under the right costal margin in a subhepatic position. Gently lift the liver and then quickly let it go. This lifting is performed differently depending on the ligament upon which you are concentrating. For the coronary ligament, place your fingers on the middle of the liver and push posterosuperiorly. For the left triangular ligament, place the fingers to the left of the midline (as with stomach manipulation) and push the liver posterosuperiorly and to the left. For the right triangular ligament, place the fingers on the right extremity of the liver and lift it posterosuperiorly and to the right. This technique should be repeated 3-4 times at the site of the problem. Recoil is particularly useful for a "frozen" liver which has lost its motility.

INDIRECT TECHNIQUES

Indirect manipulation can be performed on three planes, using the ribs. For manipulation on the *frontal plane,* with the patient in the supine position, place yourself on his right, with your right hand on the right lateral costal margin and your left hand fixing the right shoulder. Push the bottom right ribs in the direction of the umbilicus until you reach the limit of costal elasticity *(Illustration 5-5).* You can then treat either

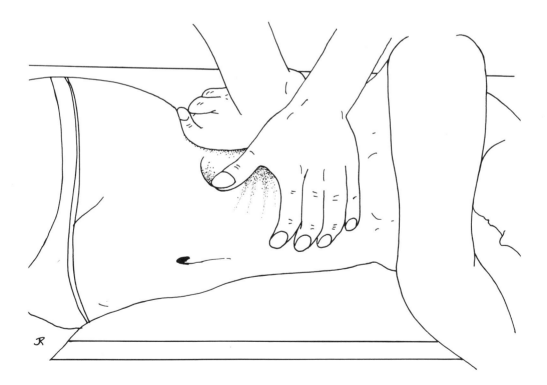

Illustration 5-6
Transverse Compression of the Liver (Lateral Decubitus Position)

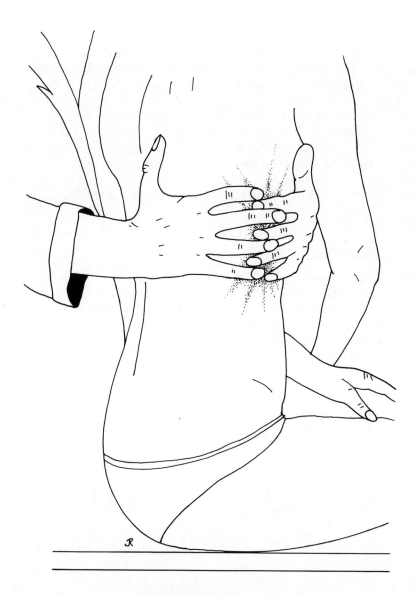

Illustration 5-7
Transverse Compression of the Liver (Seated Position)

by pulling the costal margin toward yourself while grasping the edge of the liver in your hands, or by letting the ribs come back suddenly in recoil. Before applying this technique, mobilize the ribs several times to gain elasticity and to engage the mechanoreceptors. At the end of manipulation, combine the costal maneuver with stretching of the arm in order to increase the stretching effect of the hepatic attachments on the diaphragm and pleurae.

For a variation with the patient in the left lateral decubitus position, place yourself behind him with the table in a low position (adjustable-height tables certainly increase our efficiency). Push the bottom ribs toward the umbilicus as with the supine variation. This very efficient technique can also be performed with transverse compression *(Illustration 5-6)*. You work with your body weight. For a third variation, with the patient seated, seat yourself to his left with your hands around and compressing the right inferior aspect of the thorax *(Illustration 5-7)*. The advantage of this technique is that it permits the mobilization of the lateral plane of the liver (which is often restricted after hepatitis) on the ribs.

For indirect manipulation of the liver in the *sagittal plane*, with the patient in the lateral left decubitus position with legs bent, position yourself behind the patient. Place your left hand behind the right ribs, facing the posterosuperior part of the liver, while the right hand is on the front of the body, facing the anteroinferior part of the liver (the positions of the hands can be reversed). Your hands will function synchronously, one pushing the ribs and liver anteroinferiorly and the other serving as a fixed point. To add recoil to this technique, wait until the hand which is mobilizing anteroinferiorly is at its maximal extent. With the other, push the ribs posterosuperiorly and then, simultaneously, release both hands *(Illustration 5-8)*. In a variation on this technique, the patient is in the seated position with hands clasped behind the neck. Place your right palm on the posterior angles of the ribs which protect the liver. With your left hand, lift the patient's elbows, bringing the vertebral column and ribs into backward bending while

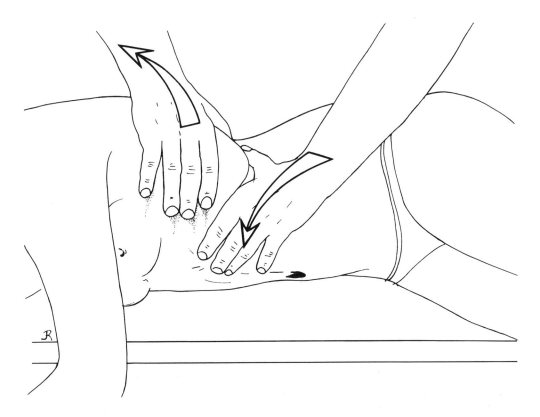

Illustration 5-8
Indirect Manipulation of the Liver (Sagittal Plane)

pushing the posterior part of the ribs anterosuperiorly. This technique permits stretching of the posterior attachment zones of the liver, as well as the diaphragm, pleurae and costal cartilages.

Indirect manipulation of the liver is also possible in the *transverse plane*, with the patient in the left lateral decubitus position. This technique consists of pushing the ribs in a superior rather than inferior direction. In order to successfully take the ribs and liver with you, place both thumbs on the posterior part of the right ribs *(Illustration 5-9)*. This movement is harder to perform but is an important addition to your repertoire. It strongly engages the liver attachments, particularly the left triangular ligament. For a variation in the seated position, take up the patient's elbows with one hand in order to bring the upper limbs, ribs and vertebra into left rotation. The other hand, applying left costal pressure, serves to increase the stretching.

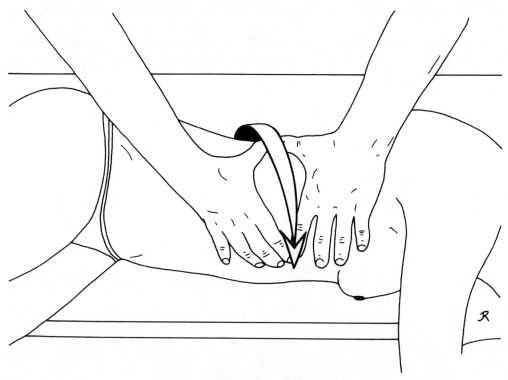

Illustration 5-9
Indirect Manipulation of the Liver (Transverse Plane)

COMBINED TECHNIQUE

With the patient in the supine position, maintain the right side of his thorax against the table and bring the bent lower limbs into left rotation. Alternatively, with the patient in the left lateral decubitus position, use one hand to stretch the right arm posterosuperiorly. With the other hand, push the lower right hemithorax downward and, only afterward, toward the xiphoid process *(Illustration 5-10)*. This is also an excellent form of stretching for the diaphragm and pleurae.

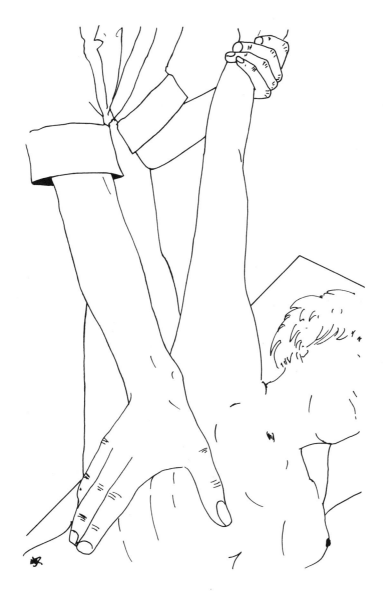

Illustration 5-10
Combined Manipulation of the Liver (Lateral Decubitus Position)

INDUCTION

General induction can be performed with the patient in the seated position. I like this technique because my hands are directly on the liver and the whole body works with me. Apply hepatic subcostal pressure with the fingers, and proceed with the general induction technique (chapter 1). The patient's body will move around the liver. This whole-body technique will free restrictions (if present) of the right kidney, pyloric region, hepatic flexure, extrahepatic bile ducts, lesser omentum, etc.

TREATMENT STRATEGY

Treatment of the liver should begin with hepatic lifting techniques which mobilize all the liver attachments and enable you to directly evaluate the hepatic tissue. After 5-6 mobilizations, follow up with recoil and techniques which free the extrahepatic bile ducts, as described in chapter 6. Retest all the articulations of the liver. If a serious restriction persists, focus on releasing it, and the others will free themselves. Do not forget the lower limbs.

Initial attention to freeing the fasciae and other supporting structures will always enhance the efficiency of hepatic induction, as well as cranial techniques. Restrictions of the right parietal, temporal, and sphenoid bones are sometimes associated with those of the liver.

Recommendations

Be wary of cervical or subclavicular adenopathies. If these exist, always refer the patient for appropriate evaluation. In a patient who shows hepatic problems without known infection, the observation of hepatomegaly in association with splenomegaly and a hard, irregular and painful liver necessitates immediate referral to an oncologist.

Benign hepatic injury, on the other hand, is an indication for osteopathic treatment, which will in most cases produce positive results when applied systematically. Because this type of problem is extremely common, we have our work cut out for us!

Some patients are hypersensitive to the presence of sulfites used for preserving certain foods (cider, beer, whiskey, fish, seafood, fast foods, sauerkraut, chips, canned mushrooms, various fruits and vegetables, etc.). Sulfites can cause migraines, urticaria, conjunctivitis, food intolerance, and a variety of other (sometimes puzzling) symptoms. Help your patients to be aware of these possibilities. Sulfites are commonly used, and potentially toxic to the liver and gallbladder, yet many people know nothing about them. A sensible diet associated with appropriate manipulation of the liver, gallbladder, and bile ducts brings good results for problems due to hepatic malfunction, including those affecting the skin.

Chapter Six:
The Gallbladder and Bile Ducts

Table of Contents

The Gallbladder and Bile Ducts

I am devoting a separate chapter to the gallbladder and bile ducts because, in spite of their close anatomical and physiological relationships to the liver, their pathology often affects the body in different ways. Functional problems of the gallbladder are common, and frequently show psychological or emotional causes and effects. This organ has the role of accepting overflow in all senses of the word. One could almost say that in some cases a spasm or inflammation of the gallbladder can be a beneficial response in terms of the whole body.

For me, gallbladder problems are similar to duodenitis in that they may not appear serious in the beginning, but must be carefully watched as they can lead to the development of ulcers. A prolonged pathology of the bile ducts can have serious consequences on hepatic integrity. Some disorders which affect both the liver and gallbladder were discussed in the previous chapter.

Physiology and Anatomy

The gallbladder has a capacity of about 33 ml. It stores bile which is produced in the liver, and regulates its passage into the duodenum via the common bile duct. The gallbladder is partially peritonized, which may explain its sensitivity and mobility. The cystic duct which empties the gallbladder is curved, 3-4 cm long, and has a diameter of 3-4 mm. It joins the common hepatic duct from the liver to form the common bile duct, which in turn joins the pancreatic duct to enter the duodenum via the duodenal papilla (sometimes called the ampulla or papilla of Vater). The sphincter of Oddi regulates passage of bile through the duodenal papilla.

In order to manipulate the gallbladder effectively, you should be familiar with the orientation of its body, which is from front to back, from left to right, and from bottom to top *(Illustration 6-1)*. It is necessary to follow this oblique axis closely in order to obtain good results. Otherwise, your treatments may have an adverse effect.

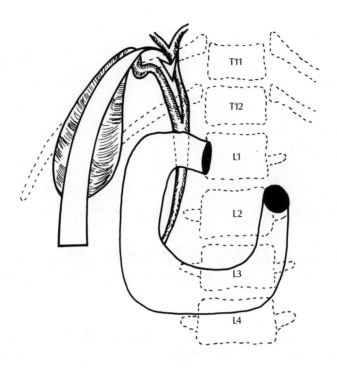

Illustration 6-1
Orientation of the Gallbladder

In adults, the surface projection of the gallbladder is on an imaginary line connecting the umbilicus to the right nipple or mid-clavicle, at its intersection with the costal margin. However, in children it is much more medial. The gallbladder has a variety of anatomical relationships which can lead to restrictions and disruption of proper function *(Illustration 6-2)*.

Sympathetic innervation of the gallbladder is from the celiac ganglion, and innervation of its peritoneal surface from the phrenic nerve. Sensory nerves of the gallbladder and bile duct, which can produce a sensation of pain, are stimulated by the tension existing in the walls of these structures. Contraction of smooth muscle in the wall depends on the vagus nerve, i.e., biliary excretion is under parasympathetic control. Secretion of bile in the liver is controlled by the hormones secretin, gastrin and cholecystokinin (CCK).

The gallbladder concentrates the bile salts and pigments it receives from the liver as much as 40-fold. Half an hour after the appearance of chyme in the duodenum, release of CCK, in combination with gastric and vagal reflexes, causes emptying of the gallbladder. On average, 15 ml of bile are released by contraction of the gallbladder. This contraction increases the pressure in the common bile duct, opening the sphincter of Oddi. Normally, pressure in the pancreatic duct is higher than that of the common bile duct.

The state of the gallbladder depends greatly upon the individual's psychological status. In particular, when a person is upset upon receiving bad news or seeing an accident, the body's first reaction is often an intense contraction of the gallbladder (less often the stomach). With repetition, this phenomenon can lead to inflammation. This correlation between the psyche and gallbladder applies primarily to superficial psychological tensions; when the problem is deeper and stronger, the entire liver reacts.

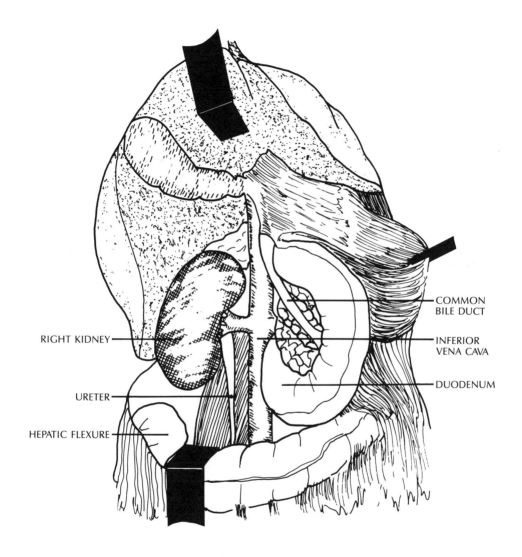

Illustration 6-2
Relationships of the Gallbladder (After Gregoire and Oberlin)

The common bile duct is 6 cm long, very wide in its upper part and becoming narrower inferiorly. It is deeply set (10-15 cm under the skin), and attached to the posterior side of the superior duodenum. This bile duct is sensitive, particularly to rapid distention. The pain fibers, as they run toward the spinal cord, are associated with the sympathetic afferent fibers. Normal, progressive elevation of pressure in the common bile duct causes only occasional vague discomfort. Pain is produced only by sudden elevation of pressure (biliary colic).

An understanding of biliary dyskinesia increases our appreciation of the conditions needed for efficient functioning of the bile ducts: a good duct system, suppleness of surrounding tissues, good tone, and good synchronization of the gallbladder with the sphincter of Oddi. These conditions will be discussed in sequence below.

Diameter of the ducts must be regular, lumen unobstructed, and the walls extensible, elastic, tonic and able to maintain longitudinal tension. As much as 1 liter of bile per day may pass through these ducts. You can achieve significant effects on this duct system, i.e., increase traction along the longitudinal axis in order to increase the parietal force of contractility, and release mechanical restrictions by removing fibroses from the fascial environment of the common bile duct, cystic duct, and gallbladder. These manipulations are performed while the organ is under traction (first longitudinal and then transverse).

PRESSURES

Mechanical problems of the gallbladder and bile ducts are hydraulic in nature. Diaphragmatic attraction, which has a major role in liver function, does not have the same effect on the gallbladder. Pressure within the bile capillaries must exceed the resistance of viscosity. Following inflammation, pressure must be even greater to overcome the added resistance of friction within the bile capillaries and the decreased elasticity of the surrounding tissues. In the intervals between periods of digestion, the resistance of biliary flow, opposed by the sphincter of Oddi, directs most of the bile toward the relaxed gallbladder.

When fasting, the pressure in the lumen of the gallbladder is only 10 cm H_2O, the equivalent of abdominal pressure. When the gallbladder contracts following a meal, its pressure is approximately 30 cm H_2O. Pressure of biliary secretion in the liver is approximately 20 cm H_2O, and that in the common bile duct 7-12 cm H_2O. The pressure necessary for crossing the sphincter of Oddi is about 15 cm H_2O. Expulsion of bile by contraction of the gallbladder is necessary to accomplish this. If there are gallstones present, they will go into the common bile duct because of this same force.

Hormonal changes are important in the processes of contraction and stone formation. For example, progesterone slows down parasympathetic motor activity and biliary evacuation, leading to the formation of stones. Rapid liquid absorption by the mucosa of the gallbladder (also under hormonal control) prevents pressure rising in the bile ducts, but also encourages the formation of stones.

Clearly, the gallbladder is not simply an inert bag that contains bile, but an active structure with important connections to the endocrine and nervous (including psychological) systems. To work efficiently, it must have soft walls that permit rapid absorption of liquids. Manipulation of the gallbladder affects not only excretion of bile, but also its other excretory functions, and pressures throughout the biliary system.

Pathology

GENERAL SYMPTOMS

I shall discuss throughout this section the symptoms of injury to the gallbladder or common bile duct in specific and well-defined pathologies. First, I would like to mention some classically-known general symptoms of injury to these organs. Recall that for ulcer sufferers, meals typically relieve the symptoms of discomfort for an hour or so. With mechanical biliary problems, malaise is likewise slightly relieved immediately after eating. Soon, however, the symptoms increase: nausea, heaviness, fine perspiration, fever, and selective aversion for certain smells and tastes (e.g., chocolate, cream, fatty foods). Other general symptoms include stale alkaline-smelling breath (ulcers or gastritis more often cause acid-smelling breath) and right retroscapular pain. A number of less common symptoms will be mentioned later in this section.

BILIARY COLIC AND OCCLUSION

These disorders involve quick and complete obstruction of bile flow by a stone, spasm, or constriction. Colic has a very abrupt onset, can last for hours, and ends fairly quickly, leaving a sensation of soreness. This distinguishes it from intestinal problems, which have a more gradual onset. Also, colic pain is not aggravated by movement, whereas pain of musculoskeletal origin often is. The most frequent cause is a stone in the cystic duct. Pain is felt in the right hypochondrium, with radiation to the right retroscapular area. There is a sensitive point facing the gallbladder, caused by inflammation of the adjacent parietal peritoneum.

Spasm of the gallbladder or common bile duct leads to sudden, tearing, transfixing attacks of pain accompanied by nausea, vomiting, abdominal distention, and pain in the right hypochondrium radiating toward the shoulders or the back. The temperature may be slightly elevated. Murphy's sign is positive for gallbladder problems. One can also consider inflammation of the gallbladder, bile ducts, or surrounding tissues including the sphincter of Oddi. There may be some difficulty in differentiating these diagnoses from:

- ulcers or stomach tumors
- acute appendicitis attacks (retrocecal or subhepatic appendix)
- acute pancreatitis (pain radiates more toward the epigastrium, left side of the thoracolumbar column, and left sacroiliac joint)
- right renal colic or any right kidney problems accompanied by urethral pain, pain along the path of the genitofemoral nerve, or painful, excessive, or reduced urination.

Occlusion of the lower part of the common bile duct is a rapid and severe disorder accompanied by acute epigastric pain. Bile backs up and causes distention of the tributary ducts, leading to stimulation of the visceral stretch and pressure receptors. Resulting pain may also be perceived around the right scapula or cervical vertebrae. Progressive narrowing of the common bile duct, in contrast to complete occlusion, is painless. With occlusion, jaundice will occur because concentration of conjugated and nonconjugated bilirubin increases in the blood and tissues. Other symptoms include intense itching, fatty stools, tendency to hemorrhage, fever, and chills. In 75% of cases, bile duct infection (cholangitis) is the origin of the problem.

GALLSTONES

This is an extremely common disorder. In the United States 8% of men and at least 20% of women over the age of 40 are affected by gallstones, and 2 million cholecystectomies are performed every year. Following the cutting of the vagus nerve to the stomach (abdominal vagotomy), gallstones increase because of massive elimination by the gallbladder, which shares the same innervation. Therefore it is very important to monitor activity of the bile ducts in ulcer patients who have undergone this operation. Gallstones are usually made up of calcium bile salts and cholesterol. Mechanisms of stone formation are not well understood. In vitro, the center of an artificial stone can form in as short a time as a few hours.

Possible causes of stone formation include:

- excess of non-soluble (and/or deficit of soluble) substances
- excessive concentration of bile in the gallbladder, with stasis
- disturbed afferent nerve stimulation, spasms of the bile duct wall, or too great a parietal thickening
- a fibrosed or scarred visceral environment (as may follow an ulcer); the scarring fixes the antropyloric region and duodenum, and contributes to pressure imbalances between bile capillaries
- age, because saturation of bile with cholesterol increases until middle age. Frequency of stones is twice as high in women below 50 vs. those above 50.

There have been many studies of the factors which contribute to gallstone formation, but conclusions have been highly variable. At puberty, as ovarian function begins, the concentration of cholesterol in bile increases. Estrogen-based birth control pills, and estrogen itself, increase the cholesterol saturation of bile. Thus, incidence of gallstones increases for women on the pill or toward the end of pregnancy. My clinical experience has shown that use of oral contraceptives leads to biliary excretion problems, associated with acne, overactive sebaceous and sweat glands, dermatitis, greasy hair, etc. Diabetes also increases the likelihood of stone formation.

Symptoms and Complications

Symptoms of gallstones are similar to those of biliary colic. Pain may be absent, or occur mainly in the initial stage, or be severe and accompanied by chills and fever. Utilization of imaging techniques has demonstrated that many people carry enormous stones without realizing it. The gallbladder simply becomes nonfunctional, but without outward symptoms. Migraine headaches sometimes occur during a gallbladder attack. On the other hand, some migraines have no connection with gallstones, but are due to hiatal hernia or diverticulosis.

Symptoms of stones in the common bile duct include epigastric and thoracic column pain, transitory and moderate jaundice, fever, continuous chills, and vomiting. Sometimes intestinal bacteria (e.g., E. coli, Streptococcus) are found in the gallbladder. The patient appears generally healthy apart from symptomatic attacks. When stones are present in the common bile duct, the gallbladder is typically fibrosed and non-distensible, a clear indication for osteopathic treatment.

Possible complications of gallstones include acute or chronic cholecystitis (see below). Chronic cholecystitis is a scleroinflammatory condition of the gallbladder walls where they attach to the omentum or adjacent organs. Symptoms of acute cholecystitis follow a well-established order (in 24-36 hours) of pain, fever, and jaundice. Stones in the common bile duct can bring about pancreatitis or, more rarely, cholangitis, liver abscess, cirrhosis, empyema (accumulation of pus in an organ), or even fistulization or obstruction of the intestine.

In the case of an obstruction of the common bile duct, one finds either a large dilated gallbladder or a small contracted gallbladder *(Illustration 6-3)*, depending on whether the obstruction was produced by a tumor of the pancreatic head or by a biliary stone. This is because the common bile duct does not have a subduodenal portion, while the terminal portion of the hepatic duct is behind the duodenum. If the obstruction results from a pancreatic tumor *(Illustration 6-3, left)*, the common bile duct is blocked at the terminal end and bile accumulates in the gallbladder, which becomes distended. If there is a stone in the subduodenal portion of the hepatic duct, bile cannot reach the gallbladder. Because the organ is then nonfunctional, it contracts *(Illustrations 6-3, right)*. Also, when there is a stone in the bile duct the gallbladder is usually scarred and therefore does not become distended.

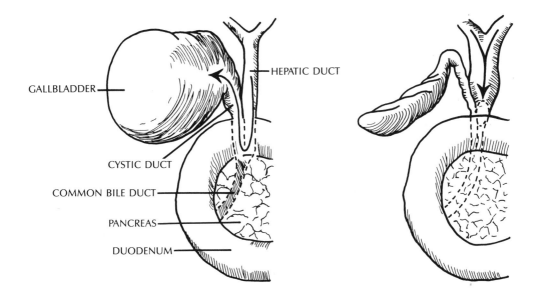

Illustration 6-3
Obstruction of the Common Bile Duct (After Testut)

This phenomenon is known as Courvoisier's law after a French surgeon (1843-1918) who stated that a dilated gallbladder in a jaundiced subject without biliary colic is likely to result from a neoplastic obstruction of the common bile duct (usually carcinoma of the pancreatic head).

CHOLECYSTITIS

Acute

Acute cholecystitis, in 95% of cases, results from a stone located in the cystic duct. The other 5% of cases are due to trauma or effects of surgery. The severe distention of the gallbladder which occurs in this disorder interferes with normal circulation and lymphatic drainage, allowing the proliferation of commensal (and normally harmless) bacteria.

Symptoms include intense pain of the upper right quadrant, nausea and vomiting, fever, mild jaundice, muscular guarding, and pain upon listening and palpation. Sometimes symptomatology is moderate, with only a vague pain of the right shoulder. When there is intense epigastric pain with definite jaundice, a stone is almost certainly present. In 50% of cases one can palpate a sensitive mass comprising the distended gallbladder and adhering omentum.

Murphy's sign is pathognomonic for gallbladder dysfunction. It is performed in the following manner: press just below the right costal margin at the midclavicular-umbilical line (the surface projection of the gallbladder) and have the patient breathe in deeply. An increase of pain accompanied by a sudden holding of the breath is a positive Murphy's sign which signifies a problem with the gallbladder.

Differential diagnosis: Colic pain is perceived low down, does not block respiration and does not radiate upward, but more toward the lumbosacral region and sacroiliac articulations. The pain of cholecystitis may be confused with that of myocardial infarction, ulcer, pancreatitis, pneumonia of the right inferior lobe, acute nephritis, renal colic, or intestinal occlusion. I must emphasize that cancer of the gallbladder presents no particular symptoms. Be particularly wary of cases with generalized signs of toxicity such as malaise, fever, loss of appetite, weight loss, jaundice, and dark and scanty urine.

Chronic

Chronic cholecystitis presents as repeated episodes of acute cholecystitis, the mucosa and smooth muscles of the gallbladder being replaced by fibrous tissue. There are frequently adhesions with neighboring structures. The ability of the gallbladder to concentrate bile is impaired. Symptoms of chronic cholecystitis are the same as those of acute cholecystitis, but often with only a slight fever.

I am no longer surprised when I encounter gallstone patients who have undergone surgical removal of the gallbladder without notable improvement of their symptoms. The actual stone is not always of great physiological significance, and may not explain all the symptoms. Sometimes, after surgical intervention, the patient feels even worse. Possible explanations include incomplete surgery, residual stones of the common bile duct, other disorders of the gallbladder or bile duct, asymptomatic neoplasm, fistula, etc. Surgical trauma can cause narrowing of the bile ducts or sphincter of Oddi; the former condition can also result from anatomic abnormality.

OTHER DISORDERS

Biliary cirrhosis is a serious complication of stones arising from negligence on the part of the patient or practitioner, or a missed diagnosis. It is a form of cirrhosis marked by prolonged jaundice due to chronic retention of bile and inflammation of the bile ducts. Hepatic fibrosis is reversible at the beginning but becomes progressively irreversible. Other symptoms are intense itching, jaundice, and portal hypertension.

Acute pancreatitis will be described in chapter 7. Gallstones are a primary cause; stones with a diameter of 2 mm or less are able to cross the sphincter of Oddi.

Biliary dyskinesia refers to defects in the control of smooth muscle activity of the gallbladder or bile ducts. Normally, the arrival of the bolus in the duodenum triggers increased secretion of CCK, which causes the gallbladder to contract and relaxes the sphincter of Oddi. There are three major types of biliary dyskinesia, all fairly common: evacuation problems (dyskinesia), tone problems (dystonia), and problems of coordination between the gallbladder and sphincter of Oddi (dyssynergia). Nausea, headache, vertigo, diarrhea and constipation are the principal symptoms. There seems to be a clear psychological component to these problems, since they are more common in anxious people. Dietary aggravating factors include alcohol, chocolate, cream, fatty foods, and various medicines. My observations indicate that biliary dyskinesia is also associated with hormonal factors, e.g., high estrogen level.

Cancer of the gallbladder is an insidious cancer found mostly in women over 70 years old. Symptoms include constant pain and a palpable mass in the right upper quadrant, general fatigue, weight loss, and jaundice. This is a relatively rare form of cancer and is usually inoperable by the time it is diagnosed.

Cancer of the bile ducts affects mostly the common bile duct and is slightly more prevalent in men 40-60 years old. Symptoms include progressive jaundice, absence of pain, itching, weight loss, and absence of bile in the stools.

Rarely, biliary obstructions result from parasitic infestations such as ascariasis and schistosomiasis, or from hydatic cysts.

LESS-COMMON SYMPTOMS

Serious biliary disorders do not require great skill or subtlety to diagnose, as they tend to make themselves obvious. However, some malfunctions are less serious, while still having the potential to detract from "quality of life." I would like you to be aware of several less-common symptoms which are sometimes of biliary origin. This list is based on my experience with thousands of patients.

- left-sided neck pain focused on the muscles which connect the transverse processes of C4-C6 (this may also reflect stomach problems because the stomach and gallbladder share common innervation)
- hypersensitivity of the left scalp and left sinus; the scalp is sensitive when the patient combs his hair
- painful tension of the left eye, frontal/nasal articulation, and/or left nostril
- difficulty with deep respiration (I suspect that irritation with inhalation occurs because the gallbladder is compressed against adjacent structures, and its sensitive peritoneal attachments are strained. On the other hand, if deep exhalation causes pain, I think more of stretching which irritates the common bile duct and extrahepatic bile ducts)
- the prone position is uncomfortable, and sleep is episodically disturbed (in contrast, a patient with hepatic problems has deep sleep of a poor quality, is tired in the morning, and takes a long time to wake up)
- general and mental fatigue are limited to the time of the attack (with liver problems, they are severe and persistent)
- hyperthermia sometimes accompanies attacks, typically between 2 A.M. and 4 A.M., whereas the patient usually feels cold upon awakening
- the patient suffers from severe non-migraine headaches, beginning on the left side and becoming generalized later during the attack

- vertigo (perhaps associated with dysfunction of the phrenic nerve or vertebral and basilar arteries)
- hypersensitivity to sulfites found in beer, cider, apple puree, chips, etc.
- the patient craves acidic foods and seasons what he eats (e.g., with vinegar, pepper, or mustard).

Diagnosis

General listening of the gallbladder is difficult to differentiate from that of the liver. The patient forward bends, along with a very slight left rotation and right sidebending. With a hepatic problem, you may notice that the patient carries out the right sidebending first and the forward bending slightly afterward. However, with a long-standing gallbladder disorder the liver itself is usually affected and the separation of the two organs becomes meaningless. For relief, the patient holds the right shoulder slightly downward and forward.

It is always interesting to observe how individuals move and hold themselves; this will usually give you the diagnosis. For example, when traveling, people who are prone to motion sickness assume this forward bending position to prevent too strong a tension on the soft tissues around the gallbladder.

PALPATION

With the patient in the supine position, palpation of the gallbladder is difficult; the seated position is preferable. The bottom of the gallbladder is more anterior and therefore more palpable. It is also easier to explore in the case of a pathology, as seen with Courvoisier's law. To carry out palpation of the gallbladder, have the patient seated and leaning forward, and apply right subcostal pressure with your right hand. Initially, place the hand at 4 fingers' width below the costal margin and move it posterosuperiorly and to the left; the precise direction will depend on the axis of the gallbladder. To avoid muscle guarding from the rectus abdominis muscle, palpate using the ulnar edge of the fingers of your right hand on the right lateral edge of this muscle.

Normally, the inferior edge of the liver is smooth and painless, whereas the gallbladder is sensitive or hypersensitive, even in people who have never had biliary problems. This demonstrates the dense innervation which characterizes the gallbladder and its peritoneal attachment. In the beginning, pay attention to this sensitivity because it is otherwise very difficult to distinguish the gallbladder from the liver.

Compress the gallbladder against the inferior surface of the liver. Severe pain, often accompanied by apnea, may signify cholecystitis. Sensitivity without intense pain is more likely to indicate a visceral spasm. It is also possible to feel fibrosis of the gallbladder walls during compression. If the sensitivity felt during compression is increased on recoil, irritation or restriction of the gallbladder walls and peritoneal attachments is indicated. Osteopathic manipulation is often effective with these conditions.

LOCAL DIFFERENTIAL DIAGNOSIS

For local differential diagnosis, place your right hand on the patient's abdomen, middle finger along the midline and palm on the umbilicus (Illustration 6-4). For dysfunctions of the *gallbladder* (arrow 1), the fingers move toward the surface projection of this organ, where the costal margin intersects the right midclavicular-umbilical line. The hand then pronates and the palm also tends to get closer to the surface projections of the gallbladder. For the *sphincter of Oddi*, the hands do not initially move upward, but directly into pronation. The thenar eminence moves onto the sphincter of Oddi, approximately 3 cm above the umbilicus on the midclavicular-umbilical line. For the *right kidney* (arrow 2), the difference is minimal; rely on the palm of the hand, which moves to the right and remains flat. The hand stabilizes itself in a position 2-3 cm to the right of the umbilicus, without moving toward the right costal margin, and then pronates.

For the *pylorus*, the hand stays on the midline and moves 7-8 cm above the umbilicus. The palm then moves to the right or left depending on the position of the pylorus. For the *liver*, the hand moves as for the gallbladder, but without pronating; the palm settles flat onto the right costal margin. For the *pancreas* (arrow 3), the hand's axis moves toward the left costal margin, creating a 30° angle with a transverse plane through the umbilicus. The thenar eminence is found on the sphincter of Oddi at the end of the movement.

INHIBITION

Inhibition techniques are useful in eliminating the possibility of an antropyloric ulcer or hepatic problem. However, they require much practice.

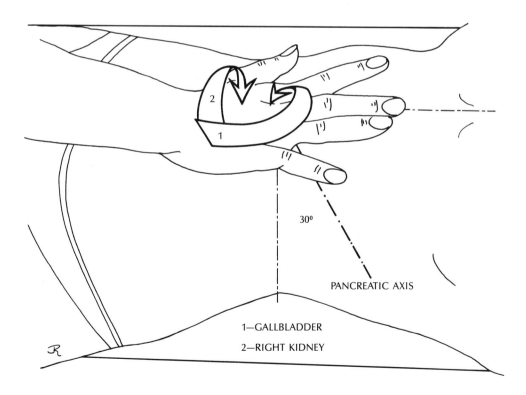

Illustration 6-4
Local Differential Diagnosis: Gallbladder

Suppose that your hand moves toward the surface projection of the gallbladder and that you wish to eliminate the possibility of antropyloric involvement. Create an inhibition point on the midline close to the xiphoid process. If your hand is still attracted toward the gallbladder point, the problem lies with this organ.

Liver involvement is usually a sign of a more serious pathology, and this possibility must also be tested. With the other hand placed flat facing the liver, inhibit hepatic motility. If the first hand is still attracted to the gallbladder point, the gallbladder itself is probably the source of the problem. If the hand no longer moves toward the right costal margin, you should suspect participation of the liver.

OTHER TESTS

Instead of compressing the gallbladder on the inferior side of the liver as described above, try stretching the tissues by putting your hands on the common bile duct (or the transverse colon which overlies it) and pushing downward. If the patient feels better, you should suspect inflammation or irritation of the gallbladder.

With gallbladder injury, lateral *compression of R9-R10* on the right disturbs inhalation. This painful disturbance may be centered on the anterior surface projection of the gallbladder. Murphy's test consists of exerting pressure on the gallbladder point in order to limit or stop respiration, as a test of significant gallbladder irritation. However, it is difficult to differentiate between the liver and gallbladder using this technique.

The common bile duct is deeply placed (15cm below the surface) behind the duodenum; I palpate it via the duodenum. It is usually not possible to differentiate it from surrounding structures. Inflammation of the common bile duct renders it sensitive to stretching, and it can therefore be tested indirectly by lifting the liver. At the end of the movement, bring the patient's thorax into backward bending to increase stretching. If bile duct inflammation is present, the patient will feel discomfort or pain between the liver and umbilicus, slightly to the right of the midline. Unfortunately, such discomfort can also result from problems of the duodenum, pylorus, or right kidney. Manipulation of the common bile duct should always be associated with that of the gallbladder, as discussed later in this chapter.

The surface projection of the *sphincter of Oddi* is found on the midclavicular-umbilical line, two fingers' width above the umbilicus. For a mobility test, place the most sensitive part of your hand (usually either the thenar or hypothenar eminence) on this point and exert pressure with a slight clockwise rotation. Sensitivity toward the end of this movement indicates a problem of the sphincter of Oddi or duodenal papilla. If the sensitivity occurs sooner, it is more likely to signify a problem of the greater omentum, small intestine, or descending duodenum. Pain on recoil following the compression suggests irritation of the local tissues. For a motility test, press the most sensitive part of your hand slightly into the point, followed by several rotations to move it in as deeply as possible. Relax the pressure a little. Normal listening to the sphincter of Oddi takes the hand into clockwise and counterclockwise rotation, with a fairly slow rhythm. If there is a problem, the palm remains flat and deep, without rotating. Local listening of a sphincter-like area that is closed or has improper motion will reveal a counterclockwise motion, in contrast to the clockwise motion present when the sphincters are open.

ASSOCIATED SKELETAL RESTRICTIONS

With disorders of the gallbladder and bile ducts, the cervical vertebrae are often restricted on the left at the level of C4-C6. I believe that these restrictions result from impaired function of the phrenic and vagus nerves. Testing of the cervical spine can help you localize biliary problems. Limited movement, with restriction of mobility more on the left side, suggests a gallbladder dysfunction. Right-sided cervical restriction is associated more with hepatic problems. Right-sided costovertebral restrictions, especially of T7-T9, are almost automatic with biliary problems. Never adjust these before you have treated the gallbladder.

The Adson-Wright test will not be positive in minor dysfunctions of the gallbladder. Positive results will be obtained with major disturbances of biliary transit which disrupt intrahepatic circulation. This test is positive with hepatic disorders because of the associated imbalance of membranous tension and blood circulation. Left and right systolic pressures, however, remain in equilibrium.

Treatment

Appropriate manipulative techniques for the gallbladder and bile ducts were discussed previously *(Visceral Manipulation,* pp. 99-107), but have since been refined and improved. Manipulation is effective for treatment of biliary stasis, gallbladder spasm, fibrosis, and even scarring and inflammation. The gallbladder is usually treated in four stages:

- restrictions are released
- the gallbladder is emptied (evacuated)
- the common bile duct is stretched
- induction (local or general) is performed.

RELEASE OF RESTRICTIONS

To release restrictions of the gallbladder, place the patient in the seated position and approach from a right subcostal position. In the case of muscular guarding, approach from the right lateral edge of the rectus abdominis muscle. Always be aware of the physiological axis of the gallbladder. Move the fingers from back to front and right to left in order to reach the anteroinferior edge of the liver. The sensitivity which is immediately triggered indicates the position of the gallbladder. Sometimes you set off the retroscapular gallbladder trigger point by being on the gallbladder. Push the fingers against the inferior side of the liver as far back as possible to get on the apex, or go underneath the gallbladder and hold it against the inferior surface of the liver. Find areas of tenderness and release them by alternately pressing slightly and relaxing them by gentle fingertip massage until the pain is relieved. After these areas have been released, i.e., ceased to be painful, make circular motions with your fingers over the area of the gallbladder. In this manner you will methodically feel the entire surface of the gallbladder and will not miss any points.

EVACUATION OF GALLBLADDER

In this stage, keep the patient in the same position and put your fingers on the apex of the gallbladder. Push rhythmically along the axis of the gallbladder to help the bile flow from apex to neck, i.e., first superomedially and then inferomedially

(Illustration 6-5). With each stroke, go just far enough to engage resistance; you will be able to go a bit farther the next time. Repeat this manipulation until it goes smoothly, usually four or five times, but never more than ten times. In thin patients you can sometimes clearly feel the neck.

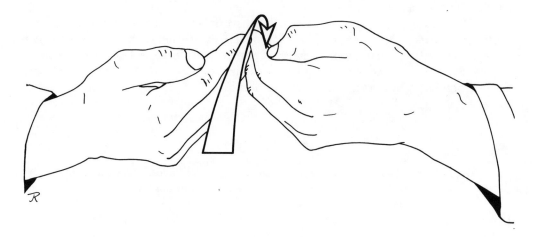

Illustration 6-5
Cholecystic Evacuation (Gallbladder Stage)

STRETCHING OF COMMON BILE DUCT

This stage begins at the moment when the fingers move downward in the direction of the sphincter of Oddi *(Illustration 6-6).* For our purposes, one could think of the common bile duct as beginning with the cystic duct. Do not relax manual pressure during this stage. To avoid triggering or increasing spasm of the gallbladder or common bile duct, your manipulation should not cause pain. When your fingers can no longer move downward, keep them in place and bring the patient into backward bending to increase the longitudinal tension of the common bile duct.

Another very useful technique is performed with the patient in the seated position with the hands clasped behind the neck. Find the sphincter of Oddi, fix it with posteriorly and inferiorly directed pressure, and stretch the common bile duct by using the elbows to backward bend and rotate the patient to the right, and slightly sidebend him to the left. Repeat rhythmically until you can feel the stretching throughout the common bile duct. A variation of this technique is to grasp the gallbladder with one hand, utilizing the subcostal approach, and push the sphincter of Oddi posteriorly, inferiorly and laterally to achieve the same effect.

GENERAL INDUCTION

Motility of the gallbladder is a see-saw motion where the gallbladder tips posteromedially (toward the midline) during expir and anterolaterally during inspir. To listen to the motility and to perform induction, place the heel of the hand on the costal margin at the level of T9. When inducing the gallbladder at the end of treatment, it is a good idea to induce the liver simultaneously, thus ensuring that they work well together.

General induction around the gallbladder is performed with the patient in the seated position. Place your fingers on the peritonized portion of the gallbladder, i.e., the middle part of the body. Usually there will be painful areas of fibrosis here. Let the body go into general induction around your hands. Initially, the patient will carry out large motions centering around the gallbladder. As usual with general induction, you should follow these large motions while simultaneously pulling your fingers in the opposite direction to stretch the fibrosed tissues. Gradually, as spasms of the gallbladder cease and the tissues become less fibrosed and sensitive, the large motions will diminish and stop.

Use this technique even if direct mobilization seems efficient to you; it mobilizes the liver and the gallbladder on all the neighboring structures and allows you to find restrictions you may not have suspected. This situation is common in cases of cholecystitis.

General induction is very useful in treating the fibrosis that usually occurs with chronic gallbladder problems. As the walls thicken, they lose their normal physiological role. Thus, the gallbladder is forced to increase its contractile pressure in order to discharge the bile. This may induce significant spasms which themselves become a problem. In 1981 my colleague Pierre Mercier and I treated a patient with cholesterosis (strawberry gallbladder with cholecystitis where the lesion consists of lipoid cells in the wall) using general induction. The thickness of the gallbladder wall was measured (with ultrasound) at the beginning of the session by Dr. Serge Cohen, and remeasured a week later. We were able to document a 50% decrease in the thickness of the wall.

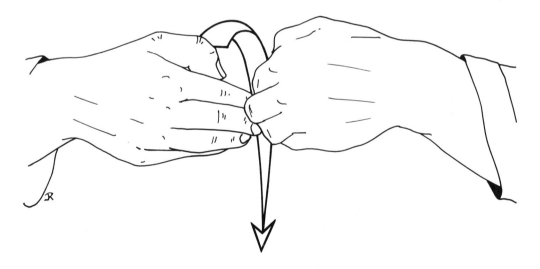

Illustration 6-6
Cholecystic Evacuation (Common Bile Duct Stage)

DIRECT TECHNIQUE

A transverse manipulation of the common bile duct can be performed with the patient in the left lateral decubitus position with the right leg bent. This is similar to the technique described for the descending duodenum. This portion of the duodenum should first be stretched to reach the common bile duct, to which it is closely linked.

Place the fingers slightly to the left of the linea alba and push them to the right and inward in the direction of the duodenum *(Illustration 6-7)*. Next, relax the pressure slightly and move the duodenum (1) transversely, (2) longitudinally toward the costal margin, and (3) longitudinally toward the umbilicus and sphincter of Oddi. These three stages result in mobilization of the length of the common bile duct.

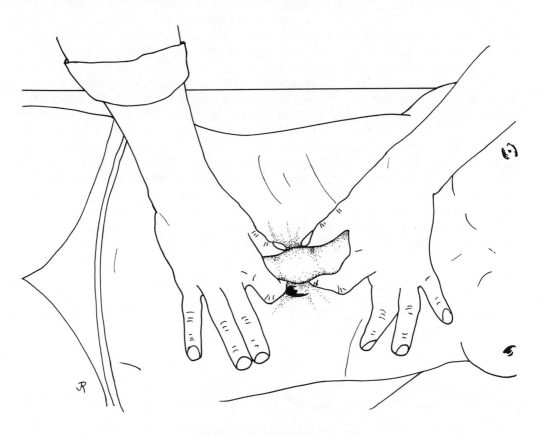

Illustration 6-7
Transverse Manipulation of the Common Bile Duct (Lateral Decubitus Position)

RECOIL

These techniques should be applied with the patient in the seated position, because by lifting the liver you stretch the common bile duct and lengthen its longitudinal axis from the liver. You can perform recoil during common bile duct stretching by pushing your fingers toward the umbilicus and quickly letting them go. The effect is concentrated on the sphincter of Oddi. You can also, during bile duct transverse manipulation as described above, "play" the descending duodenum as if it were a guitar string.

The most effective recoil is performed on the projection of the sphincter of Oddi. Push the pisiform as deeply as possible and make it slide laterally while pressing it down toward the costal margin or the ascending colon, then suddenly relax pressure. You will achieve a significant, simultaneous effect on the common bile duct and sphincter of Oddi.

TREATMENT STRATEGY

In general, I recommend that you begin with gallbladder techniques in the seated position, then proceed to the common bile duct and, lastly, the sphincter of Oddi. I have experimented by starting with the sphincter of Oddi instead, but for me beginning with the gallbladder has given better results overall. However, if your experience proves otherwise, do not hesitate to change my plan.

Stimulating the pylorus, duodenojejunal flexure, and ileocecal junction increases the effectiveness of biliary manipulation. Treatment of articular restrictions should take place only after you have systematically released those of the biliary system.

Finish the session with induction and cranial techniques. Gallbladder motility is greatly influenced by restrictions of the surrounding tissues, common bile duct, and sphincter of Oddi; these areas must therefore be treated before induction of the gallbladder. On the other hand, cranial restrictions (usually of the left frontal/temporal region, in contrast to those on the right which are more commonly due to hepatic problems) are often secondary to restrictions of the gallbladder, and induction of the gallbladder should *precede* any treatment of the cranium. This relationship is apparently due to fascial connections, to reflexes mediated by the brain centers that affect the gallbladder, and to other mechanisms which are not yet understood.

The status of all connective tissues in and around the gallbladder and bile ducts affects the tone of these biliary organs. Induction has the greatest effect on tone, notably on the spasticity of contractile fibers. A gallbladder spasm can be quickly relaxed by use of this technique. I suspect that the positive effect of articular manipulation on spasms and tone of the biliary system is mediated by the vagus nerve and celiac plexus. The reciprocal and complementary functions of the sympathetic and parasympathetic autonomic systems must be considered in this context. The interactions of these two systems are complex and often subtle; they do not always function in a simple antagonistic fashion.

The digestive system reacts to different stimuli, some mechanical (i.e., food ingestion and movement) and some involving nervous reflexes originating from reflexogenic zones (see chapter 1). In order to increase coordination between the gallbladder and sphincter of Oddi, it is necessary to manipulate not only these two organs, but also the pylorus, duodenojejunal flexure, and ileocecal junction. These areas are interdependent; if manipulation of one does not give the desired result, try the others.

Bile salts are strong choleretics (substances which stimulate excretion of bile by the liver). Thus, freeing of the gallbladder will increase hepatic secretion. Stimulation of sensory vagal nerves will also have this effect. These afferent nerves have their origins in the gallbladder and bile ducts, and can be stimulated by tension in the walls of these organs.

Hormonal Factors

I and other clinical practitioners have noted that gallbladder symptoms in women are correlated with periods of ovarian activity. Most symptoms appear in the premenstrual period, and stone formation takes place during the luteal phase. The stage of the menstrual cycle the patient is in also determines which types of manipulation are appropriate.

During ovulation, female patients often report sensitive or painful breasts, and one frequently finds middle thoracic costovertebral restrictions corresponding to mammary hyperactivity. Manipulation of the midthoracic region at this time only serves to irritate the local tissues, thereby increasing breast tenderness and spasms of the paravertebral and intercostal muscles. You could also destabilize a natural compensation that is working well for the patient. In this situation, test the costochondral articulations. If several of these are restricted and painful, avoid manipulation and have the patient return during another part of her cycle. The same is true of thoracic, lumbar and sacroiliac restrictions. I.e., if you discover such restrictions during the period of ovulation, do not treat them immediately. If you do, you run the risk of irritating an area of restriction that will probably resolve of its own accord within a few days.

For the same reason, avoid manipulating the lower lumbar and sacroiliac joints just prior to the period of menstruation. At this time, the pelvic region is congested, the uterus pulls on the sacral attachments, and all ligamentary attachments are taut and sensitive. Manipulation of, for example, the sacroiliacs, runs the risk of provoking sciatica. It is quite normal to have premenstrual restrictions in these areas. In general, when you find that all the ligamentary attachments in a particular area are sensitive, consider a hormonal or reflexogenic cause.

With men, hormonal variations (e.g., in testosterone level) are less obvious but do exist. Physical changes are less visible from the outside and are more easily overlooked. Men do have well-documented variations in sexual activity, often associated with hormonal variations.

Hormonal influence on gallbladder and bile duct function could explain disorders which the patient has observed to occur in a cyclical (e.g., monthly, equinoctial, annual) fashion. The patient may come for treatment of some secondary symptom (e.g., frequent neck and thoracic pain), and be surprised when visceral manipulation eliminates the problem. As mentioned in chapter 4, I believe that the endocrine system also has a significant role in disorders of the stomach.

Recommendations

CONTRAINDICATIONS

Gallstones are not a contraindication for osteopathy. Manipulation could conceivably cause a stone to move into the duodenal papilla, interfering with pancreatic duct function and presenting the risk of pancreatitis. However, this has never been reported, even with the thousands of gallbladder manipulations performed in France by me and others. In general, large stones do not migrate and small stones pass into the duodenum without stopping at the sphincter of Oddi.

In some cases, manipulation has been followed by serious but temporary problems such as nausea, uncontrollable vomiting, mild fever of short duration, pain around the celiac plexus, faintness, etc. In general, however, the positive results I obtained were proportional to the intensity of these temporary problems. For example, a patient in her 40s once consulted me for a problem of arterial hypertension (190/110 mm Hg). After manipulation of the gallbladder, common bile duct and sphincter of Oddi, her body became covered with petechiae (small purplish hemorrhagic spots). For one week, she experienced a rise in temperature and very pronounced fatigue. Then her blood pressure stabilized at 120/70 mm Hg, and has remained there for six years. How can one explain such reactions? The liver plays an essential role in the coagulation system through its production of heparin, prothrombin, fibrinogen, etc., but I cannot otherwise find a correlation between the treatment and the observed symptoms in this case.

If manipulation of the gallbladder or bile ducts produces major side-effects or unexpected symptoms, do not take risks. Send the patient to a specialist, or prescribe appropriate diagnostic testing. Always pay attention to general signs such as weight loss and fatigue. With development of fever, temporarily stop treatment and attempt to determine the cause of the fever. It may indicate an infection, which should not be allowed to spread in the body.

ADVICE TO THE PATIENT

Warn your patient about possible strong reactions to treatment. These include vomiting, nausea, and symptoms resembling those of depression. Fortunately, these reactions typically disappear within a few days.

Diet is important, but digestive reactions to foods depend on hormonal processes, emotional state, and extrinsic factors such as climate, country, season, etc. This helps explain the sometimes unpredictable effects of diet upon biliary function.

I must emphasize again the interdependence of the gallbladder and stomach. You may successfully treat a gallbladder disorder, only to observe the subsequent appearance of stomach pain. I believe that this phenomenon is due to their common parasympathetic innervation and reciprocal system of compensation and adaptation.

Chapter Seven:
The Pancreas and the Spleen

Table of Contents

The Pancreas and Spleen

In *Visceral Manipulation*, we did not describe any techniques for manipulating the pancreas and spleen because those in use at the time had not yet demonstrated their effectiveness. In addition, we were not sure where the techniques should be applied. Since then, I have made little progress in terms of the spleen, but somewhat more for the pancreas.

To treat the pancreas, I generally work via the sphincter of Oddi where, I believe, I am able to affect the transit of pancreatic juices via the pancreatic ducts. As mentioned in chapter 1, my techniques are most effective for viscera which have a secretory canal. My experience with hundreds of patients has convinced me that manipulation (particularly induction) does have an effect on the secretory action of the pancreas, but I have not been able to document this with either laboratory tests or imaging techniques.

I am even farther from being able to demonstrate positive effects of osteopathic manipulation on spleen function. This organ has no secretory canals and I am far from fully understanding its physiology. I believe that stimulating the spleen can reinforce the body's immune defenses, but have been unable to document this. Nor can I draw conclusions from the sensitivity of the spleen, as it is very difficult to differentiate from neighboring structures during palpation.

However, one cannot waffle and qualify one's statements endlessly. Actually, the workings of many manipulative techniques are purely a matter of speculation. For example, there is no question that manipulating a vertebra can relieve back pain, but the mechanism of the action remains hypothetical. In conclusion, I will not state that it is impossible to manipulate the spleen, but do ask that you be appropriately modest in your claims and explanations regarding such treatment.

In this chapter, in addition to presenting what little information I have about the spleen, I will describe several diseases of the pancreas and some manipulative techniques which I have developed. The intricate relationship of the pancreas with the hepatobiliary system renders differential diagnosis very subtle, and often impossible.

Physiology and Anatomy

PANCREAS

This gland has a close relationship with the duodenum, and their manipulation is typically interrelated. The pancreas is larger in men, with an average weight of 70g and length of 18cm. It is divided into two portions by the transverse mesocolon, the submesocolic part being the most important. The head and body are essentially fixed. Because the tail is less fixed and is deeply placed, it is difficult to palpate and impossible to differentiate from nearby organs. Attached to the posterior abdominal wall next to the lumbar vertebrae, the body and tail respond to pressure on L1 and L2 at the midline.

For osteopathic purposes, one must recognize the two aspects of the pancreas: the exocrine aspect which discharges digestive fluids into the duodenum and is associated with the liver, and the endocrine aspect which releases insulin and glucagon into the bloodstream. The exocrine pancreas seems to react better to direct manipulation, while the endocrine pancreas reacts better to induction.

Innervation of the pancreas comes from the vagus nerve and celiac ganglion. The early pain of a cancer of the pancreatic head is due to malignant infiltration of tissues around the nerves, as well as increased pressures within the secretory ducts.

Attachments

As the pancreas was not described in *Visceral Manipulation*, I will briefly mention some of its attachments and urge you to obtain additional information from your anatomy books. This organ is supported by the duodenum and parietal peritoneum, which press it against the posterior abdominal wall *(Illustration 7-1)*. The body is suspended from the duodenojejunal flexure, and the tail is connected loosely to the spleen by a portion of the omentum. There is a 3cm groove on the posterior side of the pancreatic head which follows the common bile duct; this anatomic relationship is of therapeutic interest.

The head rests upon the bodies of L2 and (partially) L3, which are covered by the right crus of the diaphragm. Between these vertebrae and the pancreas is found adipose tissue enclosing the aorta, inferior vena cava, and right renal vein. In cases of pancreatic tumors, these vessels are compressed, causing edema of the lower limbs. The posterior side of the pancreas, in some individuals, appears to be retroperitoneal, while the anterior side is always peritoneal. In any case, the pancreas is functionally dependent on the peritoneum.

Secretory Canals

The pancreatic duct is located superior to the common bile duct, and the two usually unite before entering the descending duodenum. The common duct, sometimes called the ampulla of Vater, is found at the posteromedial part of the duodenum where it enters via the major duodenal papilla. The smaller accessory duct (duct of Santorini) begins at the level of the neck of the pancreas and enters the duodenum via the minor duodenal papilla, 2-3cm above the major duodenal papilla.

The pancreas can secrete 1.5-2.0 liters of digestive juices per day. In fasting periods, there is very little pancreatic secretion. In 70% of people, the common bile duct and pancreatic duct share a common canal (see above), about 5mm long, which presents the possibility of reflux in either direction. An abnormal movement of bile into the pancreas can produce destruction and lipidic necrosis of parenchymal cells. Dissolution of the necrotic cells (as verified on autopsy) occurs within 24 hours. In general, such biliary reflux into the pancreas does not occur because the pressure of the pancreatic duct is higher than that of the bile ducts. Exceptions occur during physiological dysfunctions of the cystic or common bile duct, or when pressure inside the ducts is raised by pathological processes such as cholecystitis or stones.

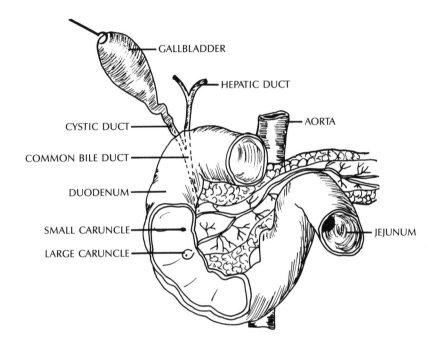

Illustration 7-1
Pancreas (After Testut)

SPLEEN

As much as possible, you should familiarize yourself with this organ so that you can detect abnormalities when they do occur. It is easy to palpate in most children, but not in adults. Easy palpation in adults indicates splenomegaly, which is a pathological sign. As noted above, the physiology of the spleen is not well understood, and I have been unable to demonstrate effects on this organ from manipulation. Is it therefore really advisable to manipulate the spleen?

Following Still's axiom that function depends on structure, it seems logical to free the anatomical environment of the spleen. We know that any mechanical restraint upsets proper visceral physiology. My recommendation is to treat the spleen indirectly via surrounding structures, e.g., the splenic flexure, stomach, diaphragm, and ribs. I have tried experimenting with direct manipulation many times, and detected little or no effect. In my opinion, therefore, such direct treatment is of questionable benefit, and could be dangerous in some situations.

The spleen is the softest and least resistant of the glandular organs. It can rupture as a result of trauma, and stitching the spleen is practically impossible. For this reason, it is often removed following trauma.

The spleen is 13 cm long, 8 cm wide and 3 cm thick in men, and generally smaller in women and older people. Its weight varies from 600 to 1,200 g. It is of a flabby consistency, its edge being narrow and presenting an inferior prolongation along the lateral edge of the left upper quadrant *(Illustration 7-2).* The parenchyma consists of two types of tissue, white pulp and red pulp, which function as part of the lymphatic and circulatory systems respectively.

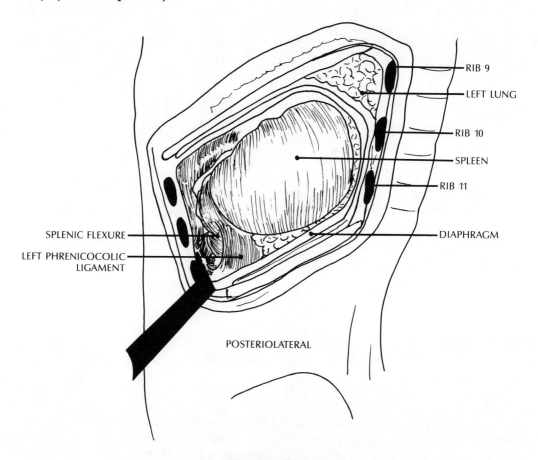

Illustration 7-2
Spleen: Posteriolateral View

Anatomic Relationships

The spleen is bounded laterally, posteriorly and superiorly by the diaphragm; medially by the posterolateral surface of the stomach; and inferiorly by the left kidney and adrenal gland, transverse mesocolon, and left phrenicocolic ligament. The left phrenicocolic ligament has a cup-shaped depression *(Testut, 1922)* in which the spleen rests, and is sometimes referred to as the suspensory ligament of the spleen. It is the only connective tissue structure capable of effectively opposing splenic prolapse as the omental connection of the spleen to the stomach and pancreas cannot really do this. The axis of the spleen is similar in direction to that of the bottom ribs, i.e., from top to bottom, back to front, and outside to inside. Spatially, the splenic compartment is delimited superiorly by a horizontal plane going through the fifth left intercostal space and the diaphragmatic dome at the height of T10; inferiorly by a horizontal plane going through the inferior edge of the rib cage, the transverse colon and its mesentery; laterally by the thoracic wall; and medially by the fundus and the greater curvature of the stomach.

Due to its relative lack of attachments, the spleen is mobile in its compartment and tends to follow the movements of the diaphragm. During inhalation, it moves downward and horizontally. When a person sits down, bends over, etc., the position of the spleen is also shifted. When the stomach is full, it is moved anteroinferiorly. Even the transverse colon, when distended, affects its position.

Functions

Since the spleen serves a blood storage function within the circulatory system, its volume and weight can vary two-fold. Due to the presence of a small quantity of contractile tissue in the white pulp, it is able to contract and release blood into general circulation. The spleen contains a considerable number of lymphocytes and functions in antibody formation; however, splenectomy does not cause a significant decrease in antibody levels. This organ is important in phagocytosis of bacteria, and of worn-out red blood cells and platelets. During embryonic life, the spleen plays an active hematopoietic role, and this function may continue or reappear later, particularly if the hematopoietic activity of the bone marrow is diminished.

Pathology

PANCREAS

Acute Pancreatitis
This is a condition that usually accompanies other pathologies, by far the most common of which are alcoholism and gallstones. It may also be found in patients with peptic ulcers, infectious diseases (e.g., mumps, hepatitis), hyperparathyroidism, and some connective tissue disorders. It can also occur secondary to trauma or certain drugs (including birth control pills, tetracycline and commonly-used diuretics).

The most widely-held theory at present for the pathogenesis of this disease is that it results from autodigestion of the pancreas by activation of proteolytic and lipolytic digestive enzymes inside the pancreas rather than the small intestine. Bile reflux into the pancreatic ducts (see above) may be responsible. In the absence of gallstones, I suspect that bile reflux may occur secondary to inflammation or fibrosis of the duodenal papillae. Pancreatitis, which is equally frequent in men and women, is usually self-limiting and subsides within one week of onset. In extreme cases, however, it can be fatal.

Pain is characteristically intense and penetrating in nature. The location of the pain depends on the retroperitoneal position of the pancreas, and the portion of the organ affected: tail (left hypochondrium), body (epigastrium), or head (epigastrium, right hypochondrium, and T10-L2 region). The pain is often more intense in the supine position, the patient obtaining relief by assuming a seated position leaning forward, legs bent and arms crossed and pressing against the epigastrium. Pain is more or less excruciating depending on the level of destruction of the gland; in many cases, it is quite mild.

Other symptoms include:

- nausea, vomiting, problems of intestinal transit, fatty stools with undigested fibers
- the patient feels exhausted, agitated and worried
- skin is moist and extremities cold
- urinary output is decreased; hypovolemic shock may ensue
- fever is absent in the beginning, later may rise to 39°C
- the epigastrium shows muscular guarding and contractions
- pain is felt on palpation, but is less severe than spontaneous pain
- bowel sounds are decreased or absent
- in approximately 20% of patients there are pleural effusions, basilar rales and other pulmonary findings, usually on the left side.

Intense pain in the locations described above is the most common sign of acute pancreatitis. Other disorders presenting the same symptom include biliary colic, myocardial infarction, gastroduodenal ulcer, mesenteric infarction, and aortic dissection. Differential diagnosis is most difficult in the case of perforation of a hollow viscera, with the contents released into the peritoneal cavity.

Chronic Pancreatitis

The early course of this disorder is often asymptomatic. It may follow slight bouts of abdominal pain or, occasionally, acute pancreatitis. In about half of the cases there is calcification along the secretory canals or (particularly in patients with a history of alcoholism) in the parenchyma of the pancreas. The acini are replaced by fibrous tissue, with metaplasia and dilatation of the secretory canals. There is an inflammatory focus with necrotic edema and deposits of calcium salts. The islets of Langerhans are preserved. Chronic pancreatitis is found with alcoholism, hyperparathyroidism, hyperlipemia, gastric surgery or, more rarely, cystic fibrosis, trauma or peptic ulcer.

Symptoms include:

- poor digestion, with undigested fatty material and muscle fibers in the stools (causing the stool to float)
- weight loss
- epigastric pain radiating posteriorly
- mild, intermittent jaundice, dyspepsia, and chronic low-grade fever.

Pain presentation is unpredictable. It may be most intense in either the right or left upper quadrants, across the entire upper abdomen, or even referred to the anterior chest.

Cancer

Pancreatic cancer, the fourth most common cause of cancer death in the United States, has a frequency 50% higher in men than in women. After 40 years of age, diabetics and smokers have the highest risk. The peak incidence is among those over 60 years of age.

Presentation includes epigastric pain plus sharp pain of the subumbilical area, with transverse and posterior radiation that is worse in the supine position. The patient feels slight relief when standing or seated with the knees between the arms. Classic symptoms are anorexia, significant weight loss and persistent jaundice (particularly with cancer of the pancreatic head). Other common signs are intense itching, dark urine, clay-colored stools, disruption of intestinal transit (diarrhea or constipation), and depression with premonition of an important disease before the actual symptoms appear. Sometimes the gallbladder is hypertrophied to the point of being palpable, a result of its attempt to protect the hepatic parenchyma from reflux. Courvoisier's law (see chapter 6) states that feeling a dilated, nontender gallbladder in a jaundiced subject can be a sign of obstruction of the common bile duct resulting from carcinoma of the pancreatic head. Death usually follows within six months of this diagnosis. Later symptoms include metastases to the liver, enlargement of the left supraclavicular lymph nodes, spleno-megaly, and abundant putty-colored stools which smell badly and are pasty, as they contain little or no bile.

Functional Disorders

So far in this section, I have described symptoms of serious or fatal illnesses of the pancreas. There are also symptoms of less serious functional problems, many resembling those of the liver:

- hypersensitivity to smells, especially heavy perfumes
- postprandial discomfort with epigastric distress, slight nausea or sweating, and impression of warmth
- postprandial fatigue (especially from high-sugar foods), diminishing with time
- left scapular irritation following a very large meal
- superficial breathing at the end of a meal and during the early stages of digestion
- upper abdominal discomfort
- slight forward leaning position
- attraction to spicy and sour foodstuffs, taken in small quantities
- discolored stools.

In conclusion, signs of pancreatic disorders are observed mostly after meals. Such disorders tend to tire the patient, and produce a musculocutaneous reflex projection mostly toward the left scapula. A "red flag" (for cancer) is weight loss combined with an easily-palpable hypertrophied gallbladder, discolored stools, dark urine, enlarged subclavicular nodes, and slight jaundice. If a patient has several of these signs, refer him to an oncologist.

SPLEEN

As noted above, a palpable spleen in an adult is not normal. Always check for splenomegaly and adenopathy. There are about 600 lymph nodes in the body, which normally are difficult or impossible to palpate. You should examine the cervical, subclavicular, axillary, and inguinal areas, and sometimes the epitrochlear, brachial and popliteal areas for enlarged nodes. In particular, the left supraclavicular nodes are often hypertrophied with neoplasms and diseases of the spleen. Abnormal sensitivity of the sternum may indicate mediastinitis or mediastinal adenopathy.

Splenomegaly

This disorder has many possible causes. I will briefly discuss those which the practitioner is most likely to encounter in his practice. Fortunately, these cases are rare. If you can feel the spleen underneath the ninth costal space on the anterior axillary line, send the patient for a thorough work-up. This condition should not be confused with an enlarged kidney or pancreatic tumor; look for fever, adenopathies and hepatomegaly as well.

MECHANICAL ORIGIN: If you are dealing with an athletic person or one who has suffered a trauma, consider a posttraumatic hematoma. Arterial blood pressure will usually be lower in this case.

ACCOMPANIED BY ADENOPATHY: These adenopathies can be mild or severe. They are found with viruses (e.g., infectious mononucleosis, toxoplasmosis), in diseases of the lymph system (e.g., lymphoma, leukemia), or in systemic connective tissue diseases (e.g., rheumatoid arthritis, lupus, sarcoidosis).

MALIGNANT ORIGIN: A large homogenous spleen may result from lymphoma, leukemia, parasitic disease, or idiopathic congestion. A large spleen with lacunae may indicate cysts, metastases, lymphoma, etc.

In my practice, I have seen only a few cases of splenomegaly, most of which were due to infectious mononucleosis. Often the symptom that led the patient to seek treatment was neck pain, originating from the cervical adenopathy which accompanies this disease. With neck pain in children and adolescents, you must check all possible areas of lymphadenopathy. This sign is usually unimportant and follows hyperactivity of the lymph nodes or hormonal dysfunctions, but is occasionally more serious.

Look for petechiae, which develop in certain forms of leukemia. In Hodgkin's disease, you may find a unilateral cervical (more rarely axillary or inguinal) adenopathy. Nodes are initially isolated and mobile (later becoming clustered and fixed), and are usually firm, resistant and painless.

"Red flags" for malignancies include splenomegaly in varying combinations with general fatigue or weakness, abdominal pain, intense paleness, hepatomegaly, or petechiae. Patients presenting with combinations of these signs should be sent to an oncologist. Rapid diagnosis may prove to be crucial in saving a person's life.

I once saw a patient suffering from Hodgkin's disease whose only symptoms were costovertebral pain (centered on T8-T10) and general weakness. He was referred by the doctor who had performed the biopsy on his nodes. On palpation, the cervical and subclavicular nodes were slightly enlarged, but the spleen was not palpable. General listening took the patient into forward bending and left sidebending. Costovertebral mobility tests showed limitation of these movements, accompanied by discomfort. However, with increase in the force of testing, there was always some mobility. In contrast, with mechanical fixations no movement is possible. I tried to feel the spleen's motility in this patient, but without success.

Diagnosis

PANCREAS

Listening

On general listening, the patient puts himself into forward bending (chin on sternum), and then into left sidebending and right rotation. I was once able to experiment with this form of listening on five pancreatic cancer patients and twelve insulin-dependent diabetics who had agreed to change the time of their insulin injection by several hours. Surprisingly, as soon as the latter patients took their insulin, listening no longer brought them into a position of forward bending. Although the sample size was small, I believe that this diagnostic technique is correct and can be utilized. In conventional medicine, the pancreatic cancer patient is described as being bent forward with the head between the knees in order to relax tensions around the pancreas. General listening often brings the patient very close to this position of relief.

Differential Diagnosis

Place the hypothenar eminence on the sphincter of Oddi, whose projection is found on the midclavicular-umbilical line two or three fingers' width above the umbilicus. The median axis of the hand, represented by the middle finger, is found on a line making a 30° angle with the transverse plane. In order to reach the *body of the pancreas,* the hand first moves posteriorly past the sphincter of Oddi and then toward the anterior left costal margin, along the longitudinal axis of the pancreas. With practice, you will feel a "see-saw" or "blotting pad" type movement, i.e., a sequential motion in which the heel of the hand moves first, then the palm, and finally the fingers. This is motion from the head of the pancreas propagating toward the tail. The hand presses mostly with the palm (which is concave) and pads of the fingers. When the fingers move deeper, the palm slightly relaxes, and vice versa. I have experimented with this local listening technique in diabetics. Prior to their insulin injection, it was easy to feel the "see-saw" motion of the pancreas. Afterwards, it was impossible. This phenomenon provides further evidence that local listening is affected by the state of the organs.

On local listening, your hand moves in deeply, and at the end of its route carries out a slight clockwise/counterclockwise rotation at the pancreatic duct which is comparable to listening of the sphincter of Oddi. This is probably because of the connection between the pancreatic duct and sphincter of Oddi. It is very difficult to differentiate between these except that the hand moves slightly toward the tail of the pancreas at the end of the pancreatic duct movement. It is easier to use osteopathic manipulation for treatment of the head than it is for the body. Local listening of the body is often positive following major childhood infections (bacterial or viral). Others have suggested that vaccinations also have this effect, but without documentation.

For differential diagnosis of the *common bile duct,* the hypothenar eminence remains on the projection of the sphincter of Oddi, but the ulnar edge of the hand moves onto a line parallel to the midline and slightly to its right. The hand then rests on its ulnar edge and moves posterosuperiorly in a clockwise rotation. This movement, which tends to make the hand move upward, allows differentiation between listening of the hepatobiliary vs. pancreatic structures associated with the sphincter of Oddi.

For the *liver*, the hand takes the same clockwise direction as for the common bile duct without going in as deeply. At the end of the movement, the palm is on the inferior costal margin. For the *gallbladder*, the hypothenar eminence leaves the projection of the sphincter of Oddi and is attracted directly (without any rotation) toward the projection of the gallbladder, at the intersection of the midclavicular-umbilical line on R8-9. At the end of the movement, the pisiform is found against the costal margin at this projection. This is different from local listening of the liver where, because of the clockwise rotation that occurs, the entire palm is against the costal margin *(see Illustration 5-2)*.

For the *pylorus*, the hypothenar eminence moves upward and stops two fingers' width below the costal margin, on the right or the left of the midline depending on the position of the pylorus. Generally, when there is a problem it is found on the right. For the *right kidney*, the hypothenar eminence slides laterally to the right 2 cm from the umbilicus, moving in deeply and slightly superiorly. At the end of the movement, the axis of the hand is close to the midline, and on an oblique axis running medially to laterally.

Inhibition

It is difficult to differentiate between pancreatic and hepatobiliary motility. Let us assume that you are undecided between a problem of the gallbladder vs. pancreatic head. Create an inhibition point on the surface projection of the gallbladder and, with the other hand, test the pancreatic/sphincter of Oddi area. If the hand initially does not move but then, with relaxing of the inhibition point, moves toward the gallbladder, a problem of the gallbladder is indicated.

You can also place the hypothenar eminence on the surface projection of the gallbladder and create an inhibition point on the pancreatic/sphincter of Oddi projection by exerting a clockwise compression and rotation on the latter projection. If the hand on the gallbladder projection stops during the pressure and then moves toward the Oddi projection when pressure is released, you can foresee a problem of the latter area. If you apply the pressure in a counterclockwise rotation, you create a restriction which renders the test useless.

Associated Skeletal Restrictions

VERTEBRAL COLUMN: With pancreatic problems there is a characteristic restriction of T9. There may also be acute back pain around T9-T11, primarily on the left. You can demonstrate the same phenomenon in an insulin-dependent person by testing the vertebral column before and after the patient has taken insulin. I have done this about ten times; the vertebral column consistently relaxes after insulin intake. It is surprising how quickly T9 frees itself. I do not know whether the mechanism is nervous or hormonal, or both. This phenomenon, however, illustrates once again that many vertebral restrictions are due purely to visceral problems. This is why I always recommend treating visceral restrictions prior to any vertebral manipulation.

SACROILIAC JOINT: This is often fixed on the left side with pancreatic problems; however, restrictions of this articulation occur for such a multitude of causes that it is not advisable to use it as a reference. The psoas muscles and sacroiliac joints are subject to frequent restrictions mainly because they are innervated by the lumbar nerve plexuses, which also serve most of the abdominal organs. For this reason, I refer to them as the body's "waste basket." For example, at least one sacroiliac joint will typically be fixed in a woman before her menstrual period; the problem quickly resolves afterwards.

LEFT GLENOHUMERAL ARTICULATION: Pancreatic problems often generate a reflex retroscapular projection on the insertion of the levator scapulae muscle. This point is usually on the left, symmetrically opposite that of the gallbladder, and can be attributed to irritation of a branch of the phrenic nerve. A left scapular point usually signifies injury to the pancreatic body; when there is no retroscapular projection of a gallbladder problem a point on the right can indicate a problem of the exocrine pancreas. I have not been able to show a positive Adson-Wright sign or difference of arterial pressure with pancreatic problems, perhaps because the soft tissues are not affected enough to cause fascial tensions or reflex effects on the subclavian arteries.

SPLEEN

Percussion

Localize the area of splenic dullness near R10 at the back of the mid-axillary line, in front of the vertebral column. This zone is often disturbed by air contained in the stomach, or splenic flexure of the colon. Note any variation in the area of dullness. According to Bates (1980), one can also detect a slight splenomegaly by percussion of the last (usually ninth) intercostal space on the left anterior axillary line, which should normally remain tympanic even after deep inhalation.

Palpation

As with the liver, I prefer the seated position with the subcostal approach. Place your fingers on the splenic flexure and move them superolaterally. With a thin patient, where the spleen is easier to approach, ask him to slightly inhale so that the spleen slides downward and inward. Be aware that during this inhalation the patient may contract the abdominal muscles and thus push your fingers away. If you feel the spleen, it will be as a mobile oval mass, between the stomach and splenic flexure. In children the spleen is usually palpable, but in adults, as mentioned previously, the simple fact of feeling it indicates that it is abnormally enlarged.

Treatment

PANCREAS

I consider manipulation of the pancreas when motility tests are abnormal and one or more of the following symptoms are present:

- laborious digestion
- white, putty-like stools containing some undigested food
- digestive intolerance or difficulty in absorbing sugar
- excessive fatigue.

In conventional medical texts there are few descriptions of functional diseases of the pancreas. In my opinion, numerous pancreatic problems are hidden behind or misdiagnosed as functional diseases of the liver, and the boundary between these two is highly variable.

An excellent indication for osteopathic manipulation of the viscera is when secretory canals or their anastomoses cannot ensure normal transit. Such disturbances to transit can be caused by fibrosis or sclerosis of the pancreatic tissues and neighboring structures, or by sclerosis of the sphincter of Oddi with resulting disruption of pancreatic or hepatobiliary secretion.

Local

Manipulation of the duodenum and sphincter of Oddi should be the first step in osteopathic treatment of pancreatic problems. As mentioned above, pancreatic secretion can be as high as two liters per day, and this liquid mass must be able to move smoothly from the pancreas to the duodenum through the various ducts and papillae.

Start out stretching the *descending duodenum* by fixing the D1-D2 angle under the liver and lifting it posterosuperiorly. Next, use lateral manipulation to make the descending duodenum move in a transverse plane. Finally, free the *sphincter of Oddi* by direct and active/passive induction techniques (see chapter 4). I would also suggest manipulating the *right kidney*, which can free the posterior part of the descending duodenum. The *peritoneal attachments* must be released as much as possible, because deep restrictions here are often the cause of visceral restrictions.

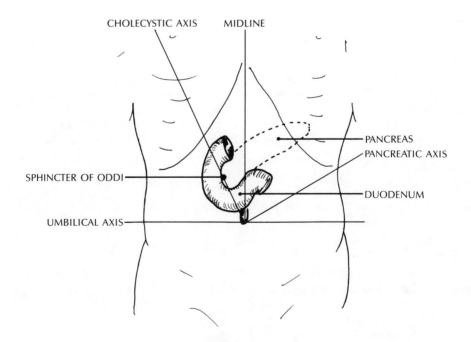

Illustration 7-3
Sphincter of Oddi and Pancreas (After Gregoire and Oberlin)

After performing several compressions/rotations of the sphincter of Oddi, perform slight direct stretching movements along the axis of the body of the pancreas, utilizing the elasticity of the tissues that lie superior to it *(Illustration 7-3)*. These manipulations must be gentle because the pancreas is a fragile organ. This is one of the reasons why I prefer mobilization of the neighboring organs rather than the pancreas itself.

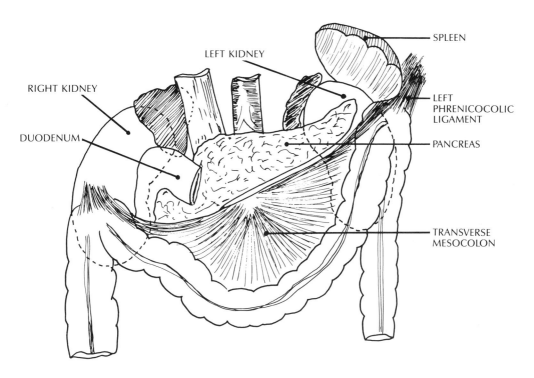

Illustration 7-4
Transverse Mesocolon and Pancreas (After Gregoire and Oberlin)

For the *body of the pancreas*, place the pisiform on the projection of the sphincter of Oddi and the remainder of the hand on the pancreatic axis (which makes an angle of 30° to the transverse plane). Then utilize a direct "see-saw" technique (see below) in which the soft tissues around the head, body and tail of the pancreas are released in sequence. Repeat this technique rhythmically until you feel a release. Finish with induction (described below), trying to include the sphincter of Oddi.

The anterior side of the pancreas is partly covered by the posterior parietal peritoneum and is crossed over by the root of the *transverse mesocolon,* to which it adheres by its inferior edge *(Illustration 7-4)*. It is important to free the transverse mesocolon by stretching it via the two colic flexures (with which it shares numerous fibers). Mobilize the two flexures superiorly and laterally. A single, superiorly directed traction is more effective for treating the ascending and descending colons, as well as Toldt's fascia. The patient sits with both hands behind the head, elbows together. With one hand, stretch a flexure superolaterally, and with the other grasp and move both of the patient's elbows to bring the thorax into rotation. In this manner, for the hepatic angle, you carry out a right rotation to stretch the phrenicocolic ligaments and transverse mesocolon.

Induction

Induction of the pancreas is performed with the heel of the hand placed over the projection of the pancreatic head, and the remainder of the hand overlying the body and tail. The technique is performed sequentially with different parts of the hand. In the beginning of expir the heel of the hand is pulled posteriorly, and as it releases, the middle of the hand is pulled down, followed by the fingers. In inspir the process begins at the fingertips and progresses to the heel of the hand. Often one phase of the cycle (either expir or inspir) will predominate. As is always the case with induction, accentuate the phase that predominates, but do not resist the other phase. Repeat the cycle until you feel a release. This type of induction is referred to as a rocking or "see-saw" technique (Illustration 7-5).

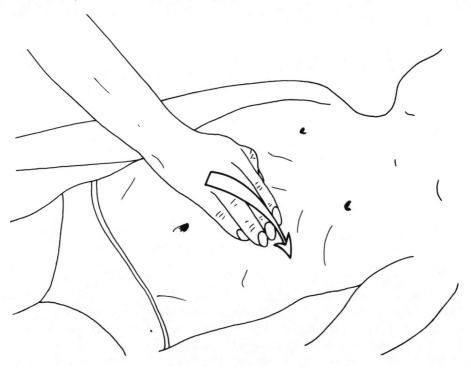

Illustration 7-5
Induction of the Pancreas

Treatment Strategy

There are few techniques which are specific for the pancreas; its position renders it interdependent with other organs such as the duodenum, transverse colon, kidneys, and spleen. Before anything else, I recommend freeing the pancreatic secretory ducts, which communicate with the hepatic bile ducts at the major duodenal papilla. Treatment should be directed next to the pancreas/sphincter of Oddi area, and then the pancreas itself, shifting progressively from direct to induction techniques. After local treatment, manipulate the liver and common bile duct, which seem to have an effect on pancreatic function. Finish treatment by eliminating spasms in highly reflexogenic zones such as the duodenojejunal flexure and ileocecal junction.

It is difficult to ascertain whether treatment of the pancreas has had an effect or not. A minor dysfunction of this organ often presents no external signs; there is nothing to listen to with a stethoscope, and imaging techniques show nothing. Thus, treatment must be based on freeing the sphincter of Oddi and normalization of listening techniques.

SPLEEN

I can offer no specific treatment for the spleen itself. You should test the mobility of neighboring organs and tissues on the principle that a fixed structure prevents the normal functioning of those organs which depend on it. Consider mobilization of the following structures:

- the left phrenicocolic ligament, upon which the spleen rests
- the transverse mesocolon, particularly its left portion which exchanges fibers with the left phrenicocolic ligament
- the left kidney, which serves to some extent as a support for the spleen, and whose prerenal fascia also shares some fibers with the transverse mesocolon and left phrenicocolic ligament
- the stomach, which is connected to the spleen by a portion of the omentum, and which can affect the spleen through variations in gastric volume.

By freeing restrictions of the structures mentioned above, you may contribute to an improvement of the spleen's physiology, but be modest in your conclusions about the efficacy of your work. As noted several times, a spleen that is easy to palpate is pathological and, like the pancreas, the spleen is quite fragile. You must therefore be especially careful and gentle in your attempts to treat this organ.

Recommendations

Never imply to a diabetic patient that the pancreatic techniques described here will eliminate the need for insulin. Manipulation of the pancreas is most effective in treating general digestive problems. Induction of this organ does affect its endocrine functions, and you may be able to significantly help adult-onset noninsulin-dependent diabetics, or allow insulin-dependent diabetics to reduce their dosage of insulin. However, these techniques are definitely incapable of completely regulating significant hyperglycemia.

Sugar is to be avoided by patients with pancreatic problems, but experience has shown that the time of ingestion is also significant. Sugar taken on an empty stomach will be most harmful. My patients have reported particularly severe problems between 11 A.M. and noon, and between 5 and 7 P.M. Foods to be avoided are listed in chapter 5.

Chapter Eight:
The Jejunoileum and Colon

Table of Contents

The Jejunoileum and Colon

In chapter 4, the duodenum was described with the stomach because their association is a clinical reality. Separation of the digestive organs for teaching purposes is always arbitrary. In this chapter, I shall consider the small and large intestines from the duodenojejunal flexure to the anus, a distance of roughly 8m. The intestinal tract is very distensible, and may appear several meters longer on autopsy than it actually is in life because of loss of tonus. I cannot describe the environment of the intestine as this would require, effectively, complete recapitulation of abdominal and pelvic anatomy. For this, please refer to your anatomy texts or *Visceral Manipulation.* Where necessary, I will emphasize certain crucial points.

In osteopathy, it is important to treat the intestinal mass because it is capable of losing its elasticity, of creating adhesions, and of going into spasm (which can last several years). After any surgical opening of the abdomen, intestinal mobility should be checked.

Physiology and Anatomy

The transverse colon is subject to diaphragmatic attraction. The hepatic and splenic flexures are suspended from the diaphragm by the phrenicocolic ligaments and are therefore, like the stomach and liver, very dependent upon the diaphragm. I previously mentioned (chapter 3) a case of migration of the splenic flexure into the thorax after a diaphragmatic hernia. The jejunoileum and sigmoid colon are less affected by diaphragmatic attraction.

PRESSURES AND ATTACHMENTS

The *jejunoileum*, attached to the peritoneal wall by the mesenteric root (which passes obliquely from the area of the duodenojejunal flexure to the ileocecal valve), behaves like a pelvic organ. Look at enteric ptoses and you will see that they begin at this line.

It is at the level of the duodenojejunal flexure that the small intestine is no longer intimately fixed to the abdominal wall and surrounding viscera. The mesenteric root contains the mesenteric vessels, lymph vessels, and lymph nodes. It is a highly reflexogenic area, and when it contains zones of abnormal tension, significant vasoconstriction may result.

The *transverse colon* is in constant motion, rising when full and descending when empty. For this reason, the organ is difficult to locate and hold. Fortunately, the transverse mesocolon, which is the part to be treated, is attached at the level of the colic flexures.

The *cecum* is a zone of mechanical conflicts, being pulled between the urogenital and digestive systems. The ileocecal junction is 4 cm wide. It acts in some ways as a sphincter, although anatomically it does not have the structure of a sphincter. Pressure on the cecal side is usually around + 20 cm H_2O in relation to that in the small intestine, and so the valve is closed. Distention of the ileum decreases this pressure differential by both mechanical and reflex means, allowing the valve to open when necessary.

The *sigmoid colon and rectum* are strongly influenced by the urogenital system. They are held by the sigmoid mesocolon, which plays a role similar to that described above for the mesenteric root. Because of its reflexogenic properties, this mesocolon should be utilized during treatment. Intraluminal pressure in the rectum can, in extreme cases, reach + 200 cm H_2O during defecation or contraction of the abdominal muscles for other reasons. Normal pressure during defecation is closer to + 50 cm H_2O. The smaller the stools, the greater the effort.

In summary, the pressure exerted on the intestinal tract ranges from -5 cm H_2O near the diaphragm to + 25 cm H_2O in the pelvic region. The mean intraluminal pressure is around + 10 cm H_2O.

REFLEXES AND DIGESTION

The hormone gastrin reinforces the gastroesophageal junction, increases gastric and intestinal motility, and relaxes the ileocecal sphincter. Manipulations of the ileocecal junction and duodenojejunal flexure are useful because they stimulate intestinointestinal, gastrointestinal and mesosigmoidal reflexes. A useful intestinointestinal reflex is the relaxation of the colon resulting from sudden distention. We can utilize this relaxation to facilitate manipulation of this organ.

The duodenojejunal flexure is sensitive to increases in luminal osmotic pressure, reduction of pH, and concentrations of glycerides and amino acids which slow down gastric peristalsis. For these reasons, this area is of great osteopathic significance. It is interesting to note that stimulation of a point in the intestine can result in contraction proximal to and relaxation distal to that point; this phenomenon can be utilized in the treatment of intestinal spasms.

Autonomic innervation of the intestines is partly via Auerbach's and Meissner's plexuses. The vagus nerve stimulates digestive activity and serves as an antagonist to sympathetic effects on the digestive organs. On the average, the colon contracts once, the duodenum twelve times, and the ileum four times per minute. It is difficult to know where a pacemaker could be when so many different rhythms are present. It is also interesting to note the similarity of the rhythm of the duodenum to that of the craniosacral system.

Mesenteric blood flow is considerable, ranging from one liter per minute at rest to four liters per minute after a meal. With limitations of cardiac output, circulation to the digestive system is reduced for the benefit of the brain and kidneys. Digestive circulation can also be disrupted by fibrosis, adhesions of attachments, or colic spasms. I believe that many functional problems result from poor digestive circulation. In such situations, symptoms would increase during digestion.

About 9 liters of water per day enter the small intestine: 1.5 liters from ingestion of liquid, and the remainder from various gastrointestinal secretions. The colon receives 0.5-1.0 liter, of which 90% is absorbed by the ascending and transverse portions. Other substances entering the proximal part of the small intestine include iron, calcium, vitamins, fats, and sugars. Major absorption sites are the jejunum (sugar, amino acids), ileum (bile salts, vitamin B12), and colon (water and electrolytes, mostly in the cecum). The colon receives 500 ml of chyme from the terminal ileum, containing undigested and nonabsorbed residues. Clearly, disorders of the intestine cannot be isolated. The general functioning of the body will be affected by such disorders, particularly that of muscles which require precisely balanced electrolyte assimilation. Spasms and tetany of muscles often originate in the intestine. Though our manipulations are local, they will have a general effect the extent of which we may not always be aware.

Pathology

Intestinal function depends on diaphragmatic mobility and intestinal peristalsis, both of which are necessary for assimilation and propulsion of chyme. With forced respiration, the colic flexures can move as much as 10 cm (normal movement is about 3 cm), which produces longitudinal tension of the ascending and descending colons. In functional colon disorders, where there are numerous spasms, stretching is limited because longitudinal tension on the colon produces pain. The body therefore prevents normal stimulation, the intestine is essentially immobilized, and there is disruption of normal digestive physiology.

RESTRICTIONS

Longitudinal tension along the ascending and descending colons occurs if there is distention of the colon and the diaphragm has normal movement. If the cecum is fixed because of scarring (due to appendectomy) of its peritoneal ligaments, this longitudinal tension is held by an inferior anchorage point, and increases gradually over time. The posterior insertion of the cecum is part of Toldt's fascia, a dense fascia covering the colon posteriorly and connecting it to the posterior parietal peritoneum. Fibrosis of Toldt's fascia produces an abnormal tension on the peritoneum, leading in turn to vascular spasms, especially of the vessels supplying the colon, small intestine, and greater omentum. Release of the peritoneum will therefore improve local circulation. Pain from restriction of the cecum is more lateral than that of the ileocecal junction.

Restriction of the cecal ligaments can have a significant effect during pregnancy. Normally, the cecum is pushed 10-15 cm superiorly by the expanding uterus. When restrictions of the cecal ligaments prevent this, tension in this area increases and can affect the kidney and genitofemoral nerve, leading to urinary difficulties, back pain, and right-sided pain of the labia majora and medial thigh.

Restrictions of the cecum often disturb sleep. There may be pain that begins at 2-3 A.M. and disappears three hours later. Patients with such problems tend to sleep on the right side with the right hip and knee flexed, and to sit cross-legged with the right knee over the left and the trunk rotated to the left. Cecal problems can also lead to knee pain. We have seen this most often in 10-14 year old girls and believe it is related to the hormonal and mechanical effects of the maturing ovaries on this area of the body, where there is already increased tension, causing pressure on the nerves that traverse the lower abdomen and innervate the knee.

Inflammation of the sigmoid colon creates inferior anchorage points of the descending colon. These points eventually limit diaphragmatic mobility and decrease the attractive effect of the diaphragm on all the abdominal organs, which thereby find their effective weight increased and begin to slide downward (see following section).

Restriction of the colon also has an effect on right renal ptoses. In such cases it is necessary, before anything else, to manipulate the liver because it adheres to the renal fascia (see chapter 9).

OBSERVATION OF THE ABDOMEN

Consider the condition of the abdominal wall, and modification of abdominal volume. Hernias, which are not always obvious, can be responsible for pain, major spasms and vascular reflex phenomena. Hernias may be found on the midline near the umbilicus, in the inguinal regions, and near post-operative scar tissue. They present the risk of a strangulated hernia. One finds either (1) a wound opening or a zone of low resistance surrounded by a fibrous ring where the finger can be inserted and where, upon exertion or coughing, the pushing of an intestinal loop can be felt; or (2) a hernia with the aspect of a small rounded mass which corresponds to a portion of the intestinal loop covered by the peritoneum. In cases of strangulation, the hernia becomes hard and incompressible, does not expand with coughing, and presents intense pain on palpation.

Always be alert for abdominal respiratory immobility with tachypnea (abnormally rapid respiration) and contraction of the abdominal wall. These may be signs of appendicitis, cholecystitis, acute pancreatitis, or subdiaphragmatic accumulation of pus. Patients with these disorders may consult you initially because of low back pain. A hard "board-like" stomach is characteristic of peritonitis. It would be surprising if someone came for consultation only after reaching this stage, but stranger things have happened.

You may observe repetitive undulating movements which are visible or palpable, and accompanied by painful spasm and distention. This phenomenon results from hyperperistalsis in response to some obstacle in the intestine; its cessation may signify complete occlusion.

We use the term "ballottement" for a procedure in which the fingers of one hand are abruptly plunged into the abdomen and held there; you will find that a freely movable mass will rebound upward. This is similar to the sensation of pushing an ice cube down into a glass and is therefore sometimes referred to in France as the "ice cube" sign. This sign may indicate either an indurated liver obscured by accumulation of serous fluid in the peritoneal cavity, or a visceral tumor with increased peritoneal fluid. When this occurs in the left iliac fossa, you may feel prominences representing fecaliths (hardened fecal material).

PROLAPSE

Prolapse of the intestine is found with:

- loss of abdominal tonus due to age or sedentary life-style
- abdominal or pelvic scarring which disturbs pressure equilibrium and visceral mobility
- any factor which decreases the tonus and distensibility of the organs and affects their attachments (see preceding chapters)
- uterine retroversion.

The latter is the major cause of intestinal prolapse in women. With retroversion, the uterus and associated structures are lowered, and the small intestine moves into the available space. Part of the small intestine moves anterior to the bladder; another part moves behind it, between the uterus and rectum. When manipulating the urogenital system, you should first disengage the small intestine.

Symptoms of intestinal prolapse are varied. The most clinically useful are:

- left abdominal pain with tenderness on palpation
- general fatigue (less severe than that from liver problems)
- belt-like back pain from T11 to L1 (greater on left side)
- patient cannot lie prone and does not like to lie on right side
- hypertonic muscle cramps with hypersensitivity of abdominal wall
- feeling of discomfort throughout the entire abdomen (with gastric prolapse there is only midline discomfort).

ABNORMAL STOOL PRODUCTION

Normal stool production is roughly 150-200g per day. There are a variety of signs and causes of abnormal function:

- hard stools accompanied by intestinal hypersecretion indicate constipation with stasis and dehydration of fecal matter
- hard stools alternating with fluid containing blood suggest an obstacle or stenosis of the descending or sigmoid colon
- putty-like, spongy or frothy stools, yellow in color, indicate problems (of pancreatic or cecal origin) of colonic fermentation, involving poor assimilation of carbohydrates
- liquid stools are often due to hypersecretion of the descending or sigmoid colon
- postprandial stools containing much partially- or non-digested food indicate a functional disorder of the gastroduodenal mucosa or liver
- greenish stools signify an excess of biliverdin resulting from biliary hypersecretion; in infants, this is the sign of acute gastroenteritis due to cow's milk
- discolored stools (putty-colored, whitish or ashen) signify a deficiency of bile pigments
- stools covered with mucus and false whitish membranes are a symptom of pseudomembranous enterocolitis
- whitish stools containing considerable fatty material indicate pancreatic or hepatic dysfunction.

Diarrhea

Chronic diarrhea is often associated with functional digestive problems. Some forms of chronic diarrhea are of infectious origins, e.g., giardiasis and dysentery, and not really within our scope, although patients may benefit from improvement of motility. Chronic functional diarrhea can usually be attributed to:

- insufficient gastric secretion
- hepatobiliary dysfunction characterized by soft, liquid postprandial stools, associated with hyperchlorhydria
- pancreatic insufficiency leading to abundant diarrhea containing excessive fatty material.

Chronic diarrhea with colitis may arise from:

- abnormal fermentation; the patient has three or four bowel movements per day; stools are of a golden yellow color, frothy aspect, and bitter smell, often preceded by painful intestinal spasm
- exaggerated fermentation of carbohydrates because of problems of the cecum, ascending and right transverse colons, accompanied by slightly malodorous nocturnal gas production
- putrefaction, from problems of the descending and left transverse colon caused by foods which are too rich in albumins; stools are infrequent, soft, brown, and of a putrid odor.

Notice the difference of smell depending on whether the problem originates in the right or left colon.

Constipation

Constipation may originate on the left or right side. Left-sided constipations are better tolerated as they are often of purely mechanical origins. Symptoms include:

- difficult defecation; fecaliths may be detected on rectal exam
- constipation of the sigmoid colon can be felt by abdominal palpation
- left colonic stases characterized by an accumulation of fecaliths in a chain along the descending colon.

Right-sided constipations are usually due to cecal stasis. Digestion continues because of the activity of anaerobic bacteria, resulting in generation of toxins and associated symptoms such as headache, anorexia, dyspepsia, bad breath, and alteration of skin color. There may also be repeated episodes of fever secondary to infection with *E. coli*. The right iliac fossa is sensitive to palpation because of cecal distention. This form of constipation is persistent, and often interspersed with periods of diarrhea.

JEJUNOILEAL DISORDERS

Diverticulosis

This is an acquired disorder which affects the mucosa and the serosa, and becomes more likely with advancing age (see "Disorders of the Colon/ Diverticulosis" below). It consists of the development of diverticula (abnormal sacs or pouches) in the intestinal wall, and may actually occur anywhere from the esophagus to the anus (in the duodenum, it usually occurs near the duodenal papilla). It has few symptoms, except when there is obstruction of the neck of the diverticulum, with diverticulitis (inflammation), hemorrhage, and necrosis of the intestinal wall.

Meckel's diverticulum is a congenital blind pouch sometimes occurring in the ileum. Found in 2% of the population (three times more frequently in men than women), it represents persistence of the omphalomesenteric duct of the embryo. It is usually found in the 50 cm segment leading up to the ileocecal valve. Check for it with obstructive syndrome (see below), which can create a palpable mass. It is manifested by slight abdominal cramps in the subumbilical region, often worsened by eating.

Obstructive Syndrome

When a smooth muscle opposes a pressure gradient, it stretches itself and then contracts firmly. This process is exaggerated and becomes painful in conditions where there is some obstacle to normal intestinal transit, e.g., tumor, occlusive gallstone (these can be up to 3 cm in diameter), annular stricture, etc. Congestion often results from loss of normal circulation. Pain is typically localized around the umbilicus and can result from mesenteric arterial insufficiency (see below) secondary to aortic degeneration. With certain problems of the diaphragmatic hiatus and gastroesophageal junction, there may be fibrosis of some fibers of the diaphragm, leading to compression of the celiac artery.

Mesenteric Arterial Insufficiency

This is a relatively rare disease, most commonly found in elderly persons and associated with vascular deficiency. It is either occlusive in nature (from thrombosis, embolism, etc.) or due to nonocclusive (heart failure, hypotension, etc.) processes. The symptoms are a dull, crampy, periumbilical pain that starts 30 minutes after meals and continues for several hours, accompanied by weight loss.

APPENDICITIS

Acute appendicitis, despite all its documented symptoms, remains difficult to diagnose. Over 1,200 appendectomies are performed every day in France. My own opinion is that many cases of appendicitis actually represent misdiagnosed mesenteric adenitis. Nevertheless, a diagnosis of true appendicitis must never be missed, or your patient will face serious consequences. This disorder is most frequent between the ages of 5 and 14, or after 55. The primary symptom is periumbilical or epigastric pain of variable intensity. In addition, there is usually anorexia, nausea, and vomiting after the onset of pain. If these signs precede the pain, you should suspect an infection (e.g., gastroenteritis or pneumonia).

Analysis of Pain

The pain is caused first (via a sympathetic pathway) by edematous distention of the serosa. Afterward, increased stimulation of the nervous system leads to the nausea and vomiting. Acute contractions of the walls of the appendix increase the pain.

Sensory innervation of the appendix is from the vagus nerve, which projects the pain onto the periumbilical area. The inflammatory process spreads gradually to the visceral peritoneum, surrounding intestinal loops, and anterior parietal peritoneum. Pain then reaches the right iliac fossa, often accompanied by constipation. Rebound tenderness with relaxation of abdominal pressure (done in a similar fashion to our recoil techniques) is only felt when the peritoneal surfaces are inflamed. A rapid diminution of pain can signify a perforation.

With normal anterior appendicitis, pain will be manifested in the lower right quadrant when the patient lifts his head against resistance. With retrocecal appendicitis, the appendix rests upon and irritates the psoas and internal obturator muscles; pain can be manifested by stretching these muscles.

Differential Diagnosis

The following disorders may be confused with appendicitis:

- inflammation of an inguinal lymph node
- inflammation of mesenteric lymph nodes (rebound tenderness is less obvious)
- gastroenteritis
- diaphragmatic irritation from a pulmonary disease
- obstruction of the appendix by a stricture
- fecaliths, worms, or a foreign body
- rupture of a graafian follicle, or ectopic pregnancy
- torsion of an ovarian cyst or testicle
- inflammation of the ovary or uterine tube (in the latter condition, mobilization of the uterine neck via vaginal insertion of a finger is painful)
- gallstones
- pyelonephritis.

Most of these conditions are accompanied by low back pain which is sometimes, at the beginning, the only symptom.

Remember the signs of peritonitis: "board-like" abdomen, intense pain on rectal examination of the peritoneum (sometimes referred to as "Douglas' shout"), and abdominal cutaneous hypersensitivity to touch.

Sooner or later you will be faced with a possible diagnosis of appendicitis. When that day arrives, the following procedure is suggested:

- palpate the painful point
- look for rigidity, muscular guarding and cutaneous hypersensitivity
- carry out abdominal recoil to manifest an acute point
- stretch the psoas and internal obturator muscles
- during rectal exam, compare pain on both sides.

Case History

I would like to describe the case of a 14 year old patient who consulted us for acute low back pain upon exertion, precipitated while serving during a tennis game. Pain was concentrated around L2, and the muscles were tense and in spasm. The lower back pain was worse with large-scale movements. Tests showed that vertebral mobility was present, despite the pain. Visceral tests demonstrated abnormal mobility and motility of the cecum. When vertebral problems are primary, there is no motion at the joint; when there is some vertebral mobility (even if pain is present), the problem usually represents the reflex manifestation of a visceral restriction. In such situations, e.g., the present case, mobility tests of the spine do not produce much pain. We deduced that when this boy served the ball, he straightened up and pulled the psoas into traction, thereby stretching the retrocecal appendix and creating an acute lumbar spasm. The parents were quite surprised when we recommended exploratory surgery; we had some difficulty persuading them. The operation revealed a retrocecal appendicitis which extended all the way to the iliac fascia and part of the right abdominal fossa.

DISORDERS OF THE COLON

Disorders of this complex organ have many possible causes and signs. You may observe abdominal distention caused by accumulation of air. Normally, the colon contains about 100 ml of gas, which may be located mostly in the flexures (if the subject is standing), transverse colon (lying down), or rectum (knee-elbow position). The colon is naturally very distensible and can adapt to variations in volume. Patients for whom gaseous distention is painful should eliminate from their diet foods such as beans, cabbage, and cauliflower that contain nonabsorbable carbohydrates, as well as milk (when there is sensitivity to lactose).

Rectal diseases can manifest themselves through modification of the rhythm of defecation, form of the stools (see "Abnormal Stool Production" above), or the presence of pus or blood in the stools. Be alert for occult bleeding, which may signify cancer of the right colon. However, melena (blackish, tar-like stools resulting from interaction of digestive juices and free blood) is rarely of colonic origin. Hemorrhages come from local lesions such as polyps, hemorrhoids, or tumors, or more generalized lesions such as colitis or hereditary telangiectasia (vascular dilatation).

During examination, palpate the colon for shrinking or gaseous distention (i.e., distal obstruction). Spasm or guarding in the iliac fossa often signifies acute diverticulitis. The rectal exam (see "Diagnosis" below) may be useful.

Analysis of Pain

Pain from colonic disorders is usually more lateral, while that from jejunoileal disorders is more central. Jejunoileal pain is often confused with that of the stomach or left kidney. Ileocecal pain, which affects the ileum as much as the cecum, is more medial than that from the cecum itself. Intestinal prolapse produces more inferior pain, radiating to the urogenital system. Sensory fibers of all parts of the colon follow sympathetic routes toward the inferior ganglia of the celiac plexus. Rectal pain is carried and projected by nerves of the sacral plexus. Colonic pain can result from distention, spasm, inflammation, or peritoneal irritation.

Diverticulosis

This common disorder involves small hernias or saclike protrusions (diverticula) of the intestinal mucosa through the surrounding muscular wall. Its frequency increases with age, and ranges between 20% and 50% in the Western population over age 50. Over 2 million people in France suffer from this disease. In 65% of cases it is found in the sigmoid colon, and never in the rectum. Diverticula are more likely to form in the sigmoid colon (which has a narrow luminal diameter and a thick layer of smooth muscle), than in the ascending colon (which is wider with a thinner muscular layer). It is more frequent in the colon than the small intestine. Deficiency of fiber in the diet is a major contributing factor. Without fiber to increase the bulk of the stools, intraluminal pressure increases, which favors formation of diverticula. Diverticulosis is often associated with varicose veins, hemorrhoids, hiatal or inguinal hernias, or gallstones. In the cul-de-sac created by a diverticulum, fecal matter stagnates and dries, creating fecaliths. Diverticula do not transform into tumors.

The disease is usually asymptomatic, but can progress to acute diverticulitis (inflammation around the diverticulum). Symptoms include fever, lower abdominal pain aggravated by defecation, and signs of peritoneal irritation (muscle spasm, guarding, and rebound tenderness). It also often results in constipation with stools of reduced size. Rectal bleeding, usually microscopic, occurs in 25% of cases. Perforation with peritonitis and sepsis can occur, especially in the infirm elderly.

Polyposis

A polyp is a structure which develops from the mucosa and projects into the lumen. Adenomatous polyps are common, particularly in elderly men whose parents were similarly afflicted. There is a great risk (50%) of malignant transformation of these polyps. The symptoms are subtle: diarrhea, manifest or occult hemorrhage, and intermittent obstruction. In 50% of patients who undergo polypectomy, new polyps appear within ten years. Polyps are found from the ileocecal junction to the anus.

Irritable Bowel Syndrome

This disorder, affecting mostly women between 15 and 45 years of age, is characterized by:

- abdominal pain along the colon
- variable bowel habits
- constipation or diarrhea
- extremely small stools (like those of goats) when spasm is strong
- relief of pain by defecation (the most common sign is constipation with pain in the left iliac fossa which is relieved by defecation)
- vasomotor instability, headache
- distention, flatulence
- middle and low back pain.

The patient is likely to be an anxious person who sweats easily, does not exhibit guarding of the abdomen, and often has a full and sensitive sigmoid colon in combination with an empty rectum. The diagnosis is supported by a long case history, lack of physical alterations, and association of the symptoms with stress. On X-ray, accented haustration and a tubulated aspect of the descending colon are observed.

We suggest that these patients limit milk, avoid laxatives, sedatives, tobacco and alcohol, and eat food which is rich in fiber. This may require some patient re-education; in France, 45 million boxes of laxatives are sold each year!

Inflammatory Bowel Disease

This term refers to inflammatory diseases of unknown origin that involve the lower intestinal tract. This disease affects both sexes equally, occurring mostly between 15 and 35 years of age. There are two forms, ulcerative colitis and Crohn's disease. The former primarily affects the colon (although there may be some involvement of the terminal ileum) and is slightly more common. Crohn's disease was originally described as just affecting the jejunoileum and is sometimes called regional enteritis. However, it can actually affect any part of the lower digestive tract and frequently occurs in the colon, sometimes without any involvement of the small intestine.

ULCERATIVE COLITIS: Symptoms include fairly sudden appearance of bloody diarrhea, abdominal pain, fever, and frequently some weight loss. If the primary site of involvement is the rectum, the patient may be constipated and complain of tenesmus. These patients often experience joint pain or changes in liver function. There may also be abnormality of the tonus and extensibility of the colon, and disappearance of haustrations or inversion of segmentation visible on X-ray. This disease carries an increased risk of colonic cancer.

CROHN'S DISEASE: As noted above, this form of inflammatory bowel disease can strike any part of the digestive system. It involves chronic inflammation affecting all layers of the intestinal wall, as well as the mesentery and regional lymph nodes. One sees shrinking of the lumen, and ulceration of the mucosa with scarring and necrotic areas which may become fistulous. This disease can disappear for years or progress in jumps. The reactivity of lymphocytes is reduced, posing a risk of inadequate intestinal immune response. Lymphocytes of the small intestine secrete immunoglobulins, particularly of the IgA subclass.

The major signs include abdominal pain (often increasing after meals), fever, poorly-formed stools or diarrhea (usually without blood), fatigue, anorexia, and sometimes back pain. When the small intestine is involved there is often right lower quadrant pain that is colicky or cramping in nature, and occasionally fistulization.

Tumors

Tumors of the colon and the rectum account for nearly half of all digestive system neoplasms and, in the United States, approximately 20% of all deaths from cancer. There is a very close relationship between such tumors and (1) adenomatous polyps (particularly where there is a strong hereditary component); (2) chronic inflammatory bowel disease (particularly ulcerative colitis). Overall, two-thirds of colonic cancers affect the sigmoid colon (more commonly in females) or rectum (more commonly in males).

Symptoms are initially non-specific, e.g., weight loss, malaise, change in bowel habits, paleness, and anemia. In cancer of the descending colon, the rhythm and size of stools is modified, and the patient has an impression of incomplete evacuation. Seventy percent of patients complain of bleeding (less commonly with right-sided tumors, as the blood becomes mixed with fecal matter). Rectal examination may show invaginations of the rectosigmoid area. With cancers of the cecum or ascending colon there is lower abdominal pain with physical activity. The cecum may be distended by fecal retention in the ascending colon. Avoid strong palpation; there is a risk of perforation.

Diagnosis can be based on:

- modification of bowel habits
- dyspepsia
- bleeding, weight loss
- presence of a mass or distention on palpation
- detection on rectal examination of vegetating or hard masses, or ulceration.

For tumors of the rectum, symptoms appear sooner: urgent or painful defecation, and even incontinence of stool. Diagnostic difficulty is common in patients with long histories of less serious intestinal disorders (e.g., irritable bowel syndrome or ulcerative colitis); they are less likely to be concerned by such symptoms.

CARCINOIDS: These are slow-growing tumors that release biologically active substances such as serotonin. They usually begin in the terminal ileum and have a tendency to metastasize to the liver without involving other organs. Primary carcinoid tumors of the appendix do not seem to metastasize, while those of the colon may metastasize but rarely have endocrine functions. The main symptoms are repeated attacks of severe flushing of the head and neck, which may or may not be accompanied by tachycardia and decreased blood pressure. These patients may develop purple telangiectasia in the same area and a plaque-like thickening of the endocardium.

Anorectal Disorders

Anorectal pain on defecation indicates anal fissures or hemorrhoids. Anorectal pain independent of defecation may indicate:

- irritation or inflammation of the anus, rectum, or sigmoid colon, characterized by tenesmus (painful tension of the rectal ampulla), with false defecation urges or intense colicky pain in the lower abdomen
- congestion accentuated by a lengthy seated position during hemorrhoidal crises
- abscesses of the anal border.

FISTULAE AND ABSCESSES: These may be associated with colitis, Crohn's disease, diverticulitis, or complications of surgery. A *fistula* is an abnormal tube-like fibrous connection from a normal cavity (especially the anal canal) to another cavity or a free surface. *Anal fissures* are superficial erosions or ulcerations of the epithelial covering of the anal canal; with this condition, defecation provokes pain which goes away in several minutes, comes back again strongly and for a long time, and finally disappears again until the next bowel movement. *Anal ulcers* result from painful spasms of the sphincter before and after defecation; they are deep and chronic. *Abscesses* produce pain that is unrelated to bowel movements and may be accompanied by fever.

HEMORRHOIDS: These are not simple varicose veins, but bunched-up masses of dilated veins in the anus or rectum, involving the local venous plexuses. Hemorrhoid thrombosis is the presence of one or several thrombotic "stones" within hemorrhoids. Such a thrombus is not likely to become an embolus (i.e., be carried off by the bloodstream to block a smaller vessel elsewhere).

Hemorrhoids may be caused by increased pressure of the portal system, pregnancy, liver disorders, increased abdominal pressure, diarrhea, tumors, or incomplete fecal evacuation. When internal hemorrhoids increase in volume, pain is not common, except in the case of thrombosis, infection, and erosion of the adjacent mucosa. Other possible symptoms include bright red bleeding and anal discomfort, and sometimes hemorrhoidal prolapse, edema, or spasm of the anal sphincter. These prolapses, which are due to lax submucosal connective tissues, can bleed and become infected. External hemorrhoids appear as a sensitive bluish swelling and are often painful.

RECTAL HEMORRHAGE: This is due to a rupture not of hemorrhoids, but of the anorectal capillaries. Ulceration due to improper use of anal thermometers or other devices is the principal cause.

ASSOCIATED PATHOLOGIES AND SYMPTOMS

A variety of reflexes and spasmodic conditions are influenced by intestinal problems. Hydronephrosis of the right renal pelvis is a major sequela to inflammatory disorders of the ileum or ileocecal junction; there is also a mechanical relationship between renal prolapse and the cecum. Many intestinal disorders are accompanied by low back pain and/or joint pain (mostly of the knees), demonstrating again that musculoskeletal pain is rarely of purely mechanical origin.

In addition to the specific and obvious symptoms listed in preceding sections, there are other symptoms which may also be related to intestinal problems:

- sensation of heaviness, or spasmodic pain, in the abdomen
- frequent emission of gas, and relief with defecation
- sensation of a full stomach; discomfort with prolonged forward bending or tight clothes
- lack of hunger
- coated tongue, bad breath
- fatigue in late afternoon and fatigue with insomnia or restless sleeping in the middle of the night
- the prone position is uncomfortable; sleep does not refresh
- stinging and light-sensitivity of eyes 3-4 hours after eating
- feet and legs feel heavy in the morning
- shallow respiration.

None of these symptoms are specific, but when associated with other symptoms or with your tests they may be significant. For some of them a mechanism can easily be proposed, e.g., fatigue is at the time of maximal intestinal activity, which is 3-8 hours after eating, depending on the speed of food metabolism; heavy feet and legs in the morning result from mesenteric venous congestion; shallow respiration is due to the colon restricting the diaphragm. However for others, e.g., stinging and light-sensitive eyes, there is a clinical correlation with intestinal problems, but no obvious mechanism.

CONCLUSION

Disorders of the large and small intestine are extremely varied in their causes, effects, and visceral relationships, since the intestines are in contact with all the other digestive organs, as well as those of the urinary and reproductive systems. Associations with other organs vary depending on the age of the individual. When one thinks of intestinal dysfunction, one often places undue emphasis on its muscular pathology; colonic spasm often originates with vascular problems. The intestine requires efficient circulatory support to ensure its proper physiological functioning. An intestinal injury inevitably has a major effect on general metabolism, and prevents satisfactory assimilation of substances which are indispensable to good muscular tonus (e.g., calcium, potassium, sodium, selenium, and vitamins).

Diagnosis

GENERAL LISTENING

With intestinal disorders, the patient always goes into forward bending, with slight variations depending on the location of the problem. For the flexures the additional movement is an almost pure sidebending, whereas for the ascending and descending colons there is more forward bending which stops at the level of the restriction and is followed by sidebending. For the hepatic flexure, the movement is finished by a slight left rotation, and for the splenic flexure by a right rotation. For the transverse colon and the superior part of the jejunoileum there is a forward bending, usually with some left rotation for the latter structure. When the inferior parts of the jejunoileum are involved, the degree of forward bending is greater and is very similar to that which occurs with bladder restrictions.

LOCAL LISTENING

In this section I will present only a brief overview of the results you may expect from differential diagnosis by local listening. Facility in this technique will require hundreds of hours of clinical practice, with confirmation of your diagnoses by other testing methods.

With the patient in the supine position, place your hand flat on the abdomen, the middle finger on the midline with the heel just superior to the umbilicus *(Illustration 8-1)*. For problems of the *hepatic flexure* (arrow 1), the hand moves obliquely superiorly and to the right in the direction of the flexure. For the *ascending colon* (arrow 2), the hand moves laterally to the right, then pronates; the index finger ends up resting on the surface projection of the ascending colon. For the *descending duodenum*, the hand pronates immediately, the index finger and hypothenar eminence coming to rest on a line parallel and two fingers' width to the right of the midline. For the *right kidney*, the heel of the hand moves to the right of the umbilicus, over the inferior pole of the kidney. For the *cecum* (arrow 3), the thenar eminence moves in the direction of the right ASIS and pronates when facing the cecum.

For problems of the *splenic flexure* (arrow 4), the movement is symmetrical with that for the hepatic flexure. At the end of the movement, the ulnar edge of the hand is on the most lateral part of the left hemithorax. By comparison, when picking up the stomach on listening, it is more central. For the *duodenojejunal flexure* (arrow 5), the heel of the hand moves to a point two or three fingers' width above the umbilicus, on the left midclavicular-umbilical line. For the *descending colon*, the hypothenar eminence

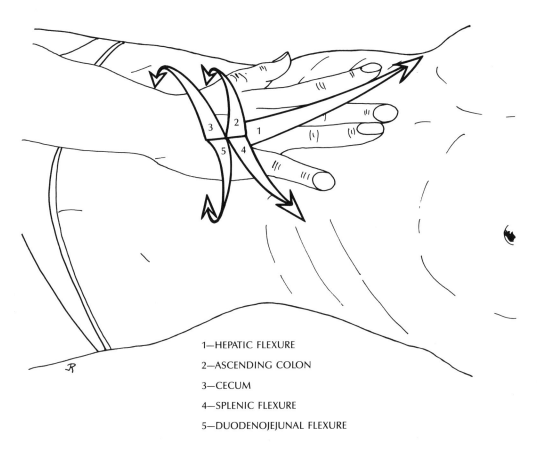

1—HEPATIC FLEXURE

2—ASCENDING COLON

3—CECUM

4—SPLENIC FLEXURE

5—DUODENOJEJUNAL FLEXURE

Illustration 8-1
Local Differential Diagnosis: Colon

moves laterally in this direction and rotates onto its ulnar edge when it gets close. For the *rectosigmoid*, the heel of the hand moves toward the left ASIS and, at the end of movement, sidebends slightly to the right.

For problems of the *jejunoileum*, the hand may move to the left or right depending on the exact location. If the entire jejunoileum is affected, the hand presses in slightly and the fingers spread out. Because the organ is so large and mobile, local listening of the small intestine is fairly difficult and requires much practice. For the *bladder and reproductive organs*, the heel of the hand remains on the midline and goes directly inferiorly toward the pubic symphysis.

INHIBITION

Let us say that, on local listening, your hand moves toward the right costal margin and you hesitate between diagnosing a problem of the gallbladder vs. the hepatic flexure. Create an inhibition point on the surface projection of the gallbladder. If your hand is still attracted by the hepatic flexure, this supports the diagnosis of a problem in this area.

Because the intestines overlap so many other organs, there are countless other opportunities for use of the inhibition technique, which I will leave to your imagination. Many examples have already been provided in preceding chapters, and the principle remains the same.

RECOIL

Sensitivity to initial palpation of the intestine indicates that the problem is localized in the organ itself; pain on recoil suggests that it will be found in the ligamentary or peritoneal attachments. Surgeons use this technique to diagnose appendicitis.

With colonic problems, the organ is sensitive, or even painful, on palpation. It may be in spasm or distended with gas. First mobilize it repeatedly until the spasms are released. Carry out a recoil technique by stretching the peritoneal attachments transversely and releasing suddenly. Sensitivity to this technique is an indication for manipulation of Toldt's fascia.

Discomfort with deep and prolonged inhalation may reflect a problem of the intestines (as they are compressed), whereas discomfort accompanying deep exhalation is more likely to indicate a problem of the attachments (which are being stretched).

RECTAL EXAM

In *Visceral Manipulation* (p. 262), we described a mobility test for the sacro-coccygeal area using the rectal route. The rectal exam can be used in osteopathic diagnosis to manifest other clinical symptoms. Fifty-five percent of adenomas are found in the rectosigmoid, and 50% of rectal cancers are within the area which can be reached by the index finger. These forms of cancer account for 10% of all gastrointestinal cancers.

Exploration should always be painless. Normally, the walls of the rectum will feel crinkled and supple. By moving the index finger toward the pubic symphysis, you may be able to feel the prostate gland or seminal vesicles in males, or the cervix or the base of the bladder in females. With retroversion of the uterus, the cervix may be felt directly anterior to the rectum. The prostate and cervix should not be tender in any way. The rectal exam may also be useful in diagnosing inflammations of the uterus, uterine tubes, ovaries, or peritoneum. Nodules in Douglas' pouch (a peritoneal sac normally lying posterior to the uterus and anterior to the rectum) may signify peritoneal metastases.

The exam can also reveal:

- anal or perianal erosion (in which case penetration of the finger causes intense pain)
- hemorrhoidal swellings, which may be more or less hardened
- the orifice of a fistula
- rectal tumors
- hardening of the wall which, accompanied by swelling, vegetating, bleeding, or painful and hardened ulcerations, suggests cancer of the anus or ampulla
- rectal shrinking, with a maximal anal diameter of 5-6 cm (this could be congenital, posttraumatic, inflammatory, or due to a tumor of the wall, or even to external compression by a neighboring tumor)
- if the glove has stool on it, check for traces of blood, tarry appearance, or a combination of blood and pus (indicating inflammation of the rectum or sigmoid colon).

ASSOCIATED SKELETAL RESTRICTIONS

Back Pain

Back pain related to the intestines is found primarily in the upper lumbar region and may come and go in association with digestive activity. Of all the visceral organs, the intestines are the most likely to be associated with acute or chronic low back pain. The intestinal smooth muscle can stay in spasm many hours and then relax for no apparent reason. With such colonic disorders, the corresponding section of the spinal cord becomes more sensitive. The threshold for the lumbar paravertebral muscles is lowered, i.e., they tend to contract easily. Acute low back pain can result from the slightest effort. Our clinical experience shows that the precipitating event is often something like, "I picked a matchstick up off the ground." Nonetheless, conventional physicians often attribute this type of pain to physical exertion, and prescribe nonsteroidal anti-inflammatory drugs. These irritate the intestinal mucosa and set up a vicious cycle, which may explain persistent low back pain in cases where no objective signs of a disc disease are present.

Sciatica

Chapter 9 will discuss etiologies of right and left sciaticas. Left sciaticas have a vascular contribution and are often accompanied by venous circulation problems affecting the rectosigmoid and lower left limb. We believe that the epidural veins which depend on the azygous system are dilated in this condition, and restrict the intervertebral foramina. One could reply that sciatica disturbs venous circulation, because the dysfunctional nerve root implies a general circulatory imbalance. For the differential diagnosis, I suggest that you perform the Lasègue test while inhibiting, with posterosuperior pressure, the rectosigmoid area. An increase of 30% in the elevation of the lower limb confirms an intestinal and perhaps vascular problem.

Right sciatica is more often of mechanical origin, usually due to abnormally high tension in the peritoneal attachments of the ileocecal junction. Test the psoas; if it is in spasm and retracted, a mechanical problem is more likely to be the cause. Use the Lasègue test by pushing the cecum posterosuperiorly and slightly medially. Again, a significant increase (more than 30%) in motion implicates the intestine.

Lower Limbs

In nearly all descriptions of intestinal pathologies (we have only covered a small part), joint pain of the lower limbs is mentioned. This connection could be explained by abnormal mechanical stimulation of the femoral nerve, or by lesional chains (see chapter 1) of the fasciae which extends in a continuous fashion between the colon, cecum, sacroiliac area, psoas muscle, iliotibial tract, and lower limbs. Chronic colon problems are often accompanied by numbness in the thighs, which varies in intensity depending on colonic rhythm and discomfort.

Think carefully when you ask questions and take histories. Some patients are preoccupied by their intestinal symptoms and overlook others, which often include ulcers, kidney dysfunctions, or (in the present context) joint pain.

Joint problems are of two types: reflex and mechanical. In the reflex type, abnormal stimulation of the nerves causes spasms and irritation of the synovial membrane or knee capsule (which is innervated by a branch of the genitofemoral nerve). Normal circulation and nutrition of the knee cartilages via surrounding tissues can be disrupted, and the capsule may be painful. In the mechanical type, an imbalance of fascial tensions causes the muscles to contract in an abnormal manner, leading to articular restriction and eventually arthritis or other degenerative conditions.

The left lower limb has a close relationship with the rectosigmoid, particularly in terms of venous circulation. You will notice that varicose veins are often found mostly on the left. This is due to the influence of the intestine and urogenital system on the venous system of the left lower limb. With the urogenital system, restrictions of the cervix also occur mostly on the left. The cervix comes to lie flat against and fixed to the rectum. Add to this the resultant rectosigmoid type of constipation and the result is a double rectal compression which is detrimental to venous circulation of the pelvis and lower limb.

Glenohumeral Articulation

In the upper limbs, one finds occasional glenohumeral periarthritis associated with intestinal problems, but less commonly than with disorders of the liver, stomach, or kidneys. This symptom is usually related to problems of the flexures and is variably painful depending upon the degree of colonic irritation. Apply the glenohumeral articulation test (chapter 1) to confirm intestinal participation; push the flexures posterosuperiorly and medially. The Adson-Wright and arterial pressure tests are rarely significant in this situation.

Treatment

The purpose of manipulation of the intestines is to free sclerosed, fibrosed and spasmodic areas, and to normalize the pressures of gases, blood, and other fluids. Although lacking any objective laboratory or imaging evidence, our clinical experience leads us to believe that we can influence intestinal metabolism and immune response. The best strategy in local treatment is to concentrate on intestinal attachments, remove fibroses, and increase elasticity. The most reflexogenic zones are the diaphragmatic attachments, mesenteric root, duodenojejunal flexure, ileocecal junction, sigmoid mesocolon, and Toldt's fascia.

HEPATIC AND SPLENIC FLEXURES

These flexures must be mobilized in all three planes to ensure the discovery of all possible restrictions.

Frontal Plane

Place yourself behind the patient, who is seated with legs hanging down, hands resting against his thighs. For the hepatic flexure *(Illustration 8-2)*, place your fingers under the ribs laterally on the right with subhepatic pressure, and move them first posterosuperiorly and medially, then anterosuperiorly and medially. Repeat this process rhythmically. For the splenic flexure, place the fingers under the rib cage laterally on the left, and carry out the same technique. We advise using recoil at the beginning of any session where the flexures are being treated; this will facilitate other techniques. Recoil

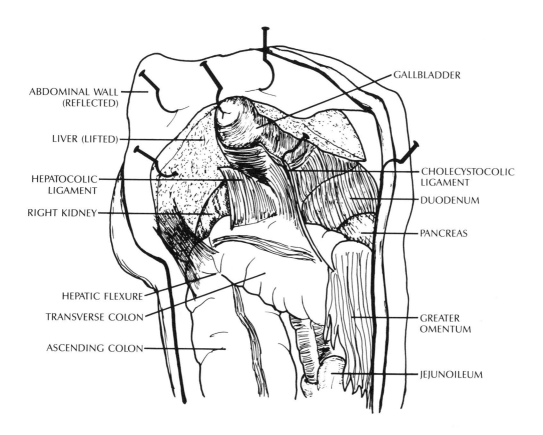

ABDOMINAL WALL
(REFLECTED)

LIVER (LIFTED)

HEPATOCOLIC
LIGAMENT

RIGHT KIDNEY

HEPATIC FLEXURE

TRANSVERSE COLON

ASCENDING COLON

GALLBLADDER

CHOLECYSTOCOLIC
LIGAMENT

DUODENUM

PANCREAS

GREATER
OMENTUM

JEJUNOILEUM

Illustration 8-2
Hepatic Flexure (After Testut)

is particularly effective in treating muscular structures such as the colon.

Alternatively, again with the patient in the seated position, fix the hepatic flexure well under your fingers, bringing it as superiorly as possible in order to exert longitudinal traction on the ascending colon *(Illustration 8-3)*. Then bring the patient into backward bending to increase stretching. In the case of a restriction of the hepatic flexure, the patient feels the fixed zones well; ask him to describe them to help you fine-tune your techniques. Recoil, releasing your hands when the longitudinal tension of the colon is at its maximum, is also very effective.

For a variation in the lateral decubitus position, the patient rests on the side opposite of that you intend to manipulate. As with the liver and stomach, you should apply the pads of the fingers of both hands subcostally, but in this case the thumbs remain back against the diaphragmatic attachments of the flexures. Push the ribs toward the umbilicus with a clockwise (on the right) or counterclockwise (on the left) motion, then either let them come back passively, or bring the costal margin toward you. This technique can also be performed by stretching the arm with one hand and, with the other, pushing the ribs to focus subdiaphragmatic stretching.

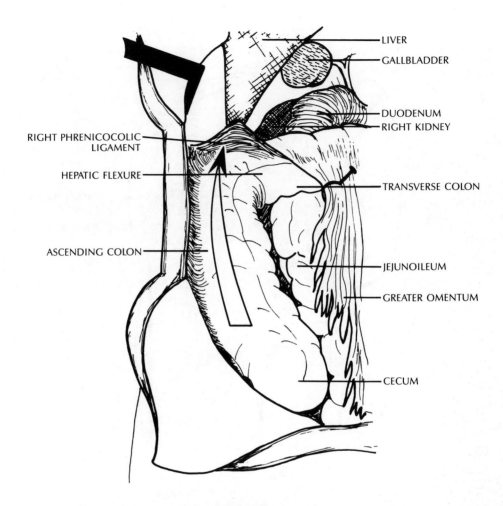

Illustration 8-3
Stretching of the Hepatic Flexure: Relationships

Sagittal Plane

The patient is again in the lateral decubitus position. Place one hand on the posterior rib cage and the other just below the anterior costal margin. Both hands act together to bring the restricted flexure medially and anterosuperiorly *(Illustration 8-4)*. For treatment of the flexures, you focus more on the vertical (superior) motion; for the liver, you use more rotation. After five or six movements, carry out recoil by releasing both hands after they have gone as far as possible.

For a variation in the seated position, the patient has both hands behind the neck. With one hand you fix the flexure posterosuperiorly behind the diaphragm. With the other, bring the patient against you with backward bending via the elbows.

Transverse Plane

The patient assumes the lateral decubitus position. Apply pressure with both hands on the appropriate costal segment, both thumbs pointing posteriorly. Push the ribs toward the xiphoid process and let them return passively. For lateral compression, put the patient in the seated position, sit beside him (opposite the side to be treated), and compress the inferior hemithorax against yourself. Release it either passively or with recoil.

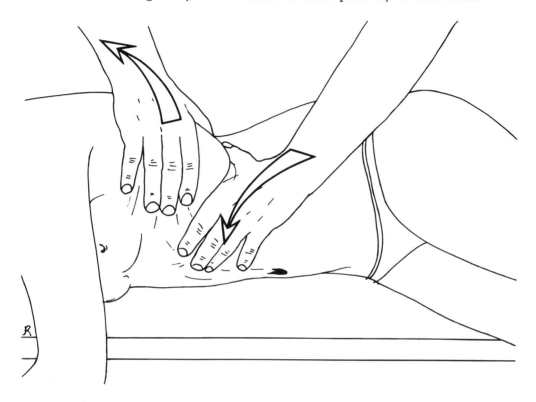

Illustration 8-4
Direct Manipulation of the Splenic Flexure (Lateral Decubitus Position)

TOLDT'S FASCIA

As previously observed, the colon can fix itself on Toldt's fascia while maintaining apparently normal superficial mobility. Such a restriction is pathogenic because it irritates the posterior parietal peritoneum and renal fascia. After locating the restriction, put both thumbs on the inferolateral part of the colon, and the fingers around the colon. Push the colon toward the midline, then release it. Use recoil prior to this treatment; this will eliminate any secondary restrictions and allow you to concentrate on the points of adhesion. This technique can be performed in the seated or lateral decubitus position.

DUODENOJEJUNAL FLEXURE AND MESENTERIC ROOT

This area *(Illustration 8-5)* is highly reflexogenic and has a significant influence on the circulatory and muscular systems of the intestine. It should be manipulated from the ends inward. The duodenojejunal flexure is symmetrically opposite the sphincter of Oddi.

With the patient in the left lateral decubitus position, place your thumbs on the medial part of the flexure to the left of the umbilicus. To reach it you must pass by the peritoneum, greater omentum, small intestine, and stomach. Manipulation takes place in an oblique superolateral direction to the left. The flexure can be brought back with the fingers, but often returns to its initial position by itself. Be sure to check the rotation of the flexure at the conclusion of this technique (which may cause it to close), and perform induction if necessary.

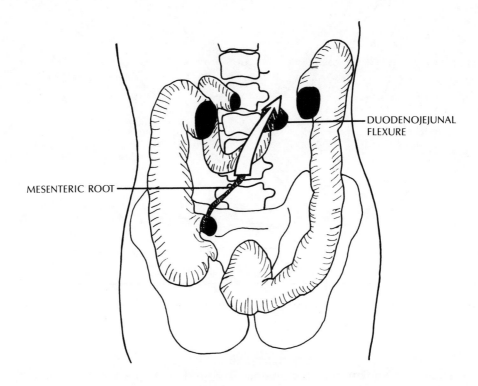

Illustration 8-5
Mesenteric Root and Duodenojejunal Flexure

For the mesenteric root, place the fingers between the duodenojejunal flexure and cecum. Move them in the direction of the posterior parietal peritoneum. To reach it, you go by the anterior parietal peritoneum, greater omentum, and loops of the small intestine. The mesenteric root should appear as a cord-like structure, which you then stretch superiorly and to the right in a direction perpendicular to its own axis. Pain on recoil often indicates an adhesion caused by infection or mechanical factors. With intestinal prolapse, the mesenteric root is sensitive and taut. Manipulate it five or six times until there is a release. Then go in less deeply and continue so that you also release the mesentery of the small intestine itself.

It goes without saying that with all these manipulations you can use recoil, but it is not enough to simply free the adhesions. Recoil is applied to the mesenteric root in a manner similar to plucking a guitar string. Put your fingers over the middle of the root, stretch it (usually toward the head), and release. Finish these techniques by combined pressure, rotation, and induction of the flexure in order to eliminate any spasm and to obtain a general reflex effect.

Finally, place the patient in the supine position and use the pressure/rotation technique which is applicable to all sphincter zones. The technique is at the same time direct and induced *(Visceral Manipulation, p. 154)*. At the end of rotation, let your palm move transversely to the left to increase the stretching effect. Recoil takes place when the limit of possible motion has been reached.

ILEOCECAL JUNCTION

Spasms or orientation problems of this area *(Illustration 8-6)* are extremely common. Because of its reflexogenic properties, this junction reacts to most forms of stress, usually by going into spasm. Orientation problems result from appendectomy or imbalance of adjacent peritoneal tensions. The imbalance creates a mechanical conflict which interferes with the passage of chyme, and may explain the numerous inflammations which appear here. In order to free the ileocecal junction effectively, you must work on its posterolateral, medial and inferior attachments. The superior ones are treated via manipulation of the colon (see above).

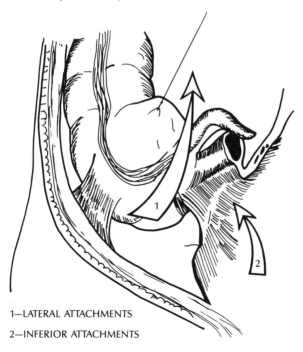

1—LATERAL ATTACHMENTS
2—INFERIOR ATTACHMENTS

Illustration 8-6
Ileocecal Junction (After Testut)

The cecum is fixed to the parietal peritoneum by ligaments or a mesentery. To treat these *posterolateral attachments,* move your fingers medially between the lateral cecum and medial wall of the ilium until you reach the restricted area. Bring the cecum in the direction of the umbilicus and let it come back again. The cecum often appears to be superficially free while still restricted at a deeper level. Failure to free a restricted cecum can render the remainder of your treatment useless.

The *medial attachments* are almost always sensitive to palpation. Place your fingers on the medial posteroinferior cecum, below the mesenteric root, and then on the medial posterosuperior part above the root. Stretch the ileocecal junction toward the right ASIS, then perpendicularly to the midline, and finally toward the tip of R12.

For the *inferior attachments*, gather up the cecum at its lowest part (lower in women) by going underneath the transverse plane passing through the superior end of the iliac bones. Be very careful not to irritate the right ovary. The approach should not be painful. Mobilize the cecum in a posterosuperior direction.

A combined technique is the most effective for releasing restrictions of the inferior cecum. Have the patient assume the knee/elbow position. Stand to his right, facing his feet. Reach around, grasp the inferior part of the cecum between the fingers and thumb of your right hand, and pull it anterosuperiorly. While maintaining this pressure, stretch the posterior attachments by extending and abducting the right leg. Repeat this smoothly and rhythmically until you feel a release.

With uncomplicated cases of constipation, we often focus on treating the pylorus and ileocecal valve. Once these are moving well (demonstrated by a clockwise rotation on local listening), the entire intestinal tract has essentially good function, and the constipation usually resolves.

We suggest that you finish treatment of the cecum with induction. This is a bit complex as the superior and inferior parts of the cecum have different motilities. The inferior cecum has a "see-saw" or "blotting paper" anterior/posterior rotation in the sagittal plane (on a transverse axis), while the superior cecum has the same motility as the ascending colon, i.e., a right/left rotation in the transverse plane (on a vertical axis). We perform induction of the cecum in two stages: first the inferior part and, only after it has released, the superior part.

SIGMOID MESOCOLON

The technique for this peritoneal attachment *(Illustration 8-7)* was previously introduced *(Visceral Manipulation*, pp. 172, 178), and I shall now complete it. Place your fingers between the left ASIS and sigmoid colon, going as far back as possible to reach the zone of peritoneal insertion. Maintain posterior pressure while moving toward the umbilicus, and then release the pressure. Repeat this process rhythmically. Next, carry out the same technique going from the pubic symphysis above the bladder. To eliminate colonic spasms, perform a recoil technique once or twice at the beginning of treatment; this will quickly release superficial and compensatory tensions. Then relax the posterior pressure so that you mobilize the actual mesocolon rather than its zone of insertion.

TREATMENT STRATEGY

Manipulate (in this order) the duodenojejunal flexure and ileocecal junction, hepatic flexure, mesenteric root, root of the sigmoid mesocolon, and local fixed zones of the colon. While this is somewhat inconsistent with our general guidelines for treating sphincter-like structures (see chapter 1, "Reflexogenic Zones"), it has in our experience been the most effective strategy.

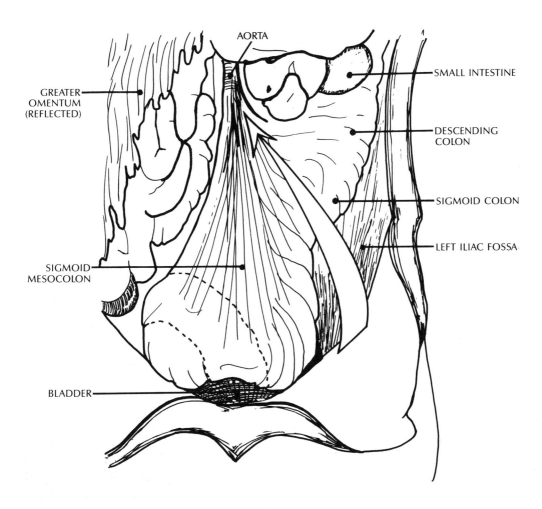

Illustration 8-7
Sigmoid Mesocolon: Direct Stretching

For a problem of the transverse colon, perform joint manipulation of both flexures. If the junctions of the jejunoileum and colon are difficult to release, release other highly reflexogenic zones (such as the sphincter of Oddi) and try again.

Recommendations

Treatment of the colon, particularly of its flexures, will obviously affect the liver, stomach, and diaphragm. Problems of the ascending and/or descending colons should make you look carefully for a possible relationship with the kidneys. The cecum is linked to the right ovary and right lower limb. The rectosigmoid has connections with the uterus and cervix in women, or the prostate gland in men. Consider its influence on the circulation of the left lower limb.

When treating the intestines, always free the large muscles (e.g., psoas, internal obturator) which insert into the abdomen. Stretching these will often release deeper zones of adhesion.

I must emphasize again the frequency of rectosigmoid cancers. Osteopaths can play an important role in the detection of such tumors because sacrococcygeal and urogenital manipulations involve frequent rectal palpation. You should be able to recognize abnormalities, and appropriately follow up "red flag" symptoms such as abdominal pain with modification of the stools or patterns of defecation, traces of blood in the stools, weight loss, or a vegetating or hardened mass felt on rectal exam.

The intestine is the organ which reflects most visibly the psychological tensions of the patient. Its frequent spasms restrict the lumbar vertebrae; however, these must not be manipulated because of the risk of creating a worse problem. For example, if there are restrictions of the lumbar paravertebral musculature due to a problem of the colon and you manipulate the lumbar vertebrae directly, you will remove a compensation created by the body. This can result in development of a more severe symptom, e.g., sciatica.

Chapter Nine:
The Kidneys

Table of Contents

The Kidneys

The kidneys are of particular importance in visceral manipulation. Renal disorders typically have wide repercussions. Being retroperitoneal, these organs are difficult to reach; their treatment therefore requires a high degree of skill. I tell my students, "Before you work on the kidneys, you had better really be *ready* to work on them."

In a healthy subject, the kidney is very difficult to feel and differentiate from surrounding structures. With practice, one learns to recognize its smooth anterior aspect. Osteopathic students often think they are palpating a kidney when they are actually around the level of the duodenum where, by pushing against the mass of viscera and peritoneal attachments, they create a "kidney" themselves. Fortunately, a kidney which requires treatment is comparatively easy to palpate because it often slides anteroinferiorly. Manipulation of the kidney nonetheless demands great manual precision.

Physiology and Anatomy

There are no fixed attachments of the kidney holding it in place *(Visceral Manipulation*, p. 192); it depends in a unique fashion upon its environment. The renal artery and vein cannot serve as an attachment because of their flexibility, and the angle they make with the inferior vena cava and abdominal aorta. The right and left kidneys are supported to some extent by diaphragmatic attraction, which presses them superiorly against the liver and colon, respectively. The right kidney is fixed somewhat by the hepatic flexure, and the left kidney to a greater extent by the splenic flexure. This renal/colonic relationship is of pathological significance, as we shall see below.

The medial edges of the kidneys are separated by 10-12 cm at the bottom and 6-7 cm at the top, which renders their oblique axis to be directed downward and laterally. The right kidney is 3.5 cm, and the left 5 cm, from the iliac crest on either side. The right and left renal fasciae are connected, providing a mechanism for shared mechanical pathologies *(Illustration 9-1)*.

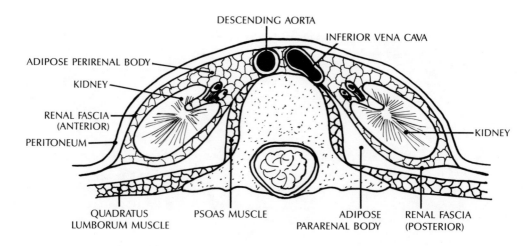

Illustration 9-1
Relationships of the Kidneys (Transverse Section)

The fascia of each kidney is divided into an anterior and posterior lamina, or layer *(Visceral Manipulation, p. 190)*. Since these two laminae are not continuous at the inferior pole of the kidney *(Illustration 9-2)*, there is a potential route for the kidney to slide downward. The anterior lamina is reinforced by Toldt's fascia where there is contact with the colon. The two laminae (which become fused above the adrenal gland) merge with the inferior surface of the diaphragm near the hiatus. Between R11 and R12, the kidneys are directly in contact with the pleural cul-de-sac. Remember that R12, depending on its length, has an extrapleural lateral third.

Between the posterior lamina and the aponeurosis of the quadratus lumborum muscle are found the twelfth intercostal, iliohypogastric, ilioinguinal, lateral femoral cutaneous, genitofemoral, and (lower down) femoral nerves. The distributions and functions of these nerves are significant in the diagnosis of renal restrictions.

Few people are aware of the magnitude of renal metabolic activity:

- each kidney contains about one million functional units called nephrons
- about 1,700 liters of blood (20-25% of total cardiac output) are sent to the kidneys via the renal artery every 24 hours
- from this, 170 liters of filtrate (devoid of cells and proteins) enter the renal parenchyma
- of this, about 99% is reabsorbed into the bloodstream, and the remaining 1-2 liters are eliminated from the body as urine.

Pathology

RENAL PTOSIS

The primary mechanical pathology of the kidneys is ptosis (or prolapse). This condition is particularly frequent in women. The female renal compartment is not as deep and thus there is more mobility of the kidney with inhalation. Our estimate is that 25% of women over 50 years of age have a renal ptosis, usually on the right. Paradoxically, some kidneys that have descended as far as the pelvis present fewer symptoms than kidneys which have undergone less drastic ptosis. This phenomenon is comparable to subluxation of a bone; most connections are broken and therefore little information can be transmitted and manifested symptomatically.

Causes and Relationships

Ptosed or fixed kidneys which have lost their mobility and motility are found more commonly on the right. The cecum and ascending colon are often causative factors. Following appendectomy, a very common operation, the cecum (which is normally fairly mobile) adheres to the parietal peritoneum laterally and posteriorly. The ileocecal junction, which sometimes loses its axis, is likewise restricted. The ascending colon loses its longitudinal mobility, and tension increases along its axis. Immobilized at

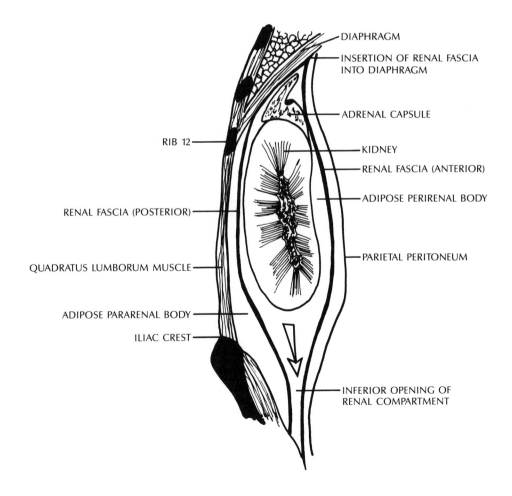

Illustration 9-2
Kidney: Sagittal Section (After Testut)

its lower end, the ascending colon pulls on its upper end, drawing the hepatic flexure downward. As noted above, the anterior lamina of the renal fascia is closely linked to Toldt's fascia, and the right kidney is thus drawn downward as well. Initially it only loses part of its mobility and motility. However, if this situation continues untreated for several years, significant ptosis inevitably results.

To illustrate the interdependence of the kidney and the cecum, take the example of chronic ileitis. The inflammation of the ileocecal region can cause hydronephrosis (abnormal accumulation of urine) in the right renal pelvis, with injury to the right ureter. To a lesser degree, minor irritation of the cecum can affect the kidney and its surrounding tissues.

The right kidney contacts the inferior surface of the liver, on which it leaves an impression. The liver, for support and mobility, depends on diaphragmatic attraction which, in turn, requires proper pleural elasticity. With various pulmonary disorders, the elastic properties of the lung and pleurae diminish, the diaphragm loses its normal tonus, the liver increases in volume, and the force of intracavitary pressure *(Visceral Manipulation*, p. 15) is reduced. The kidney is thus pushed from above by the liver and drawn from below by the cecum.

The female uterus is often retroverted, with the cervix found posteroinferiorly. The consequences of a hysterectomy are similar but more dramatic: the small intestine and some part of the colon (at least the cecum) move down to take the place of the uterus. Both of these conditions enable the mass of intestines and omenta to migrate downward. Not only does this lead to a direct downward attraction of the kidneys but, as the greater omentum is attached to the transverse mesocolon which is connected in turn to the hepatic flexure, there is pressure placed on the liver which can be transmitted to the kidneys. This is a case of renal ptosis with a colonic origin.

The left kidney, linked to the right kidney by the renal fascia, is dependent on it. However, it does not prolapse as easily. It first loses its motility, then part of its mobility, over several years. It may slide downward, but usually not very far. The lower frequency of left renal ptoses may also be due to the presence of the spleen which is smaller and therefore less likely to weigh on the kidney than the liver. In addition, scarring or other restrictions of the descending colon are rare. Left renal restrictions which do not seem impressive are, however, more poorly tolerated than comparable right renal restrictions.

Other potential causes of ptosis include:

- rapid weight loss (i.e., loss of pararenal adipose tissue)
- nervous depressions and other factors affecting basic tonus (illnesses, medicines, etc.)
- sedentary lifestyle or adverse working conditions (e.g., sitting or standing all day)
- excessive time spent traveling (e.g., in planes or cars)
- surgical intervention, with resulting abdominal atonia and scarring
- urinary infections and kidney stones, which may produce ptosis by a reflex mechanism
- colitis, because of its associated intestinal spasms, can disturb renal mobility and motility; this is often the cause of unexpected treatment failures
- intrauterine devices affect mostly left renal motility (a clinical observation without a proposed mechanism)
- trauma (e.g., chronic coughing, strong vibrations)

- certain congenital factors involving the shape of the renal compartment or unfavorable anatomical relationships (e.g., enlarged liver)
- direct traumas, particularly falls on the coccyx or ribs.

There is a strong clinical relationship between the coccyx and kidneys, although we have no satisfactory theories as to the mechanism involved. The reverse is also observed; renal manipulation, particularly on the left, can free restrictions of the coccyx.

Degrees of Ptosis

Renal ptoses can be classified into three degrees of severity. These degrees correspond to the actual anatomical course of the kidney *(Illustration 9-3)*.

FIRST DEGREE: The kidney, under various mechanical influences, begins a slight downward migration. In the process, it irritates the twelfth intercostal nerve which is between the pararenal body (the layer of adipose tissue partially surrounding the kidney), the aponeurosis of the quadratus lumborum, and the posterior lamina. The patient feels subcostal discomfort and, during the consultation, often puts his hands on the lower ribs to both explain the problem and get temporary relief. Sometimes there is sharp pain in the lower ribs, radiating toward the umbilicus. The patient cannot breathe deeply, and coughing and sneezing are very uncomfortable. The patient may come for consultation after pulmonary X-rays, the symptoms having been mistakenly attributed to a pleural problem. The hemidiaphragm over the kidney is spasmodic and less mobile, as demonstrated by a decrease in chest expansion and depth of respiration on that side.

SECOND DEGREE: The kidney continues its migration along the "rail" of the psoas. Its inferior edge becomes more anterior and its external rotation is more obvious. It begins to irritate the genitofemoral nerve and (more rarely) the lateral femoral cutaneous nerve, both of which pass through the pararenal body. The ilioinguinal and iliohypogastric nerves may also be irritated, but this seldom results in symptoms. The kidney crosses over the posterior side of the renal compartment, going obliquely downward and laterally. The patient complains of cutaneous hypersensitivity or lower abdominal pain, which can radiate toward the labia majora, pectineus muscle, ipsilateral hip, or even the lateral thighs if the lateral femoral cutaneous nerve is affected. The hyperesthesia may later give way to numbness. The results of conventional medical exams are typically negative, and the patient may be labeled as a hypochondriac. On intravenous pyelography (IVP), one can detect the external rotation of the kidney because the renal artery and vein are more visible. Tension on these vessels by this external rotation must, in our opinion, create vascular spasm. The external rotation can also stress and twist the ureter, often manifested as abdominal tension appearing about 15 minutes after drinking. We believe this can also be a factor in the development of kidney stones.

THIRD DEGREE: The kidney becomes "subluxated" and loses all contiguity with the liver or diaphragm. It begins to irritate the femoral nerve. The patient experiences hypersensitivity of the ipsilateral thigh, accompanied by pain from inflammation of the knee capsule; he may complain of knee pain with no history of trauma to the knee. The internal capsular pain increases when the knee is bent, so that kneeling or squatting positions are badly tolerated. X-ray of the knee reveals nothing, and there may be a mistaken diagnosis of arthritis.

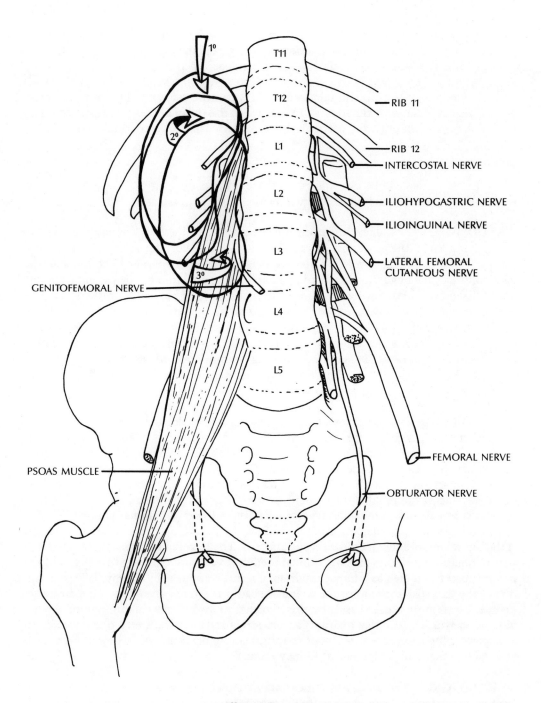

Illustration 9-3
Renal Ptosis: Three Degrees

The knee pain leads to a spasm of the psoas which tends to bring the lower leg into external rotation, with a change in its axis. Joint pain appearing in the ankle and foot becomes mechanical in nature, although visceral in origin. Initially, the articulations of the feet compensate for the mechanical imbalance and the patient may suffer repeated sprains. When the compensation by the feet is exhausted, the knee is forced to substitute, leading to sprains of the knee which are much more debilitating (it is less common to recover completely from a knee sprain).

In third degree ptosis, the inferior pole is very low and anterior ("pelvic kidney"), but the kidney is in internal rotation because it is not under the influence of the psoas. This internal rotation is better tolerated than external rotation, as it does not put so much stress on the large vessels or the ureter. Vascular spasms, when present, are usually less serious. As noted above, the third degree has fewer symptoms than the first or second, and motility may appear essentially normal.

Childbirth

During childbirth, the volume of the abdominopelvic cavity is diminished quite abruptly. Tonus and elasticity of muscles and ligaments are, in addition, altered by the effects of various hormones. If delivery is too fast, and accompanied by a heavy-handed obstetrical technique which is not synchronized with the labor, the organs are pulled downward. Certain ligamentous attachments, under too great a pressure, can even rupture. Abdominal pressure, which normally helps maintain the position of the kidneys, breaks down and contributes further to renal ptosis. Our impression is that too hasty a delivery is as harmful as too prolonged a labor.

When the kidneys of young mothers are tested, it is worrisome to note (as we have) a systematic absence of motility up to six months after childbirth. In mothers who undergo natural childbirth, the motility will return on its own after this time. Osteopathic treatment can expedite this process and may be necessary for mothers who had difficulties during labor. This decrease in renal motility is related to the loss of energy, decrease in libido, and depression often seen in new mothers.

Right vs. Left Kidney

Clinical symptoms differ depending on which kidney is involved. The right kidney can be called the "digestive kidney." In the beginning, its migration is due to effects of the liver and ascending colon. Ptosis increases intestinal problems because of the reflex spasms and direct mechanical irritations it creates. The patient complains of cecal pain similar to that of appendicitis.

The left kidney could be called the "reproductive kidney." Its restriction or ptosis affects the digestive system comparatively little, apart from a spasm of the duodenojejunal flexure, which the patient perceives as stomach pain. However, it can produce irritation of reproductive organs such as the left ovary or left spermatic cord. Clinically, we have observed an association between sexual dysfunctions and the left kidney. That is, left kidney problems affect sexual functions, and sexual problems (of various types) adversely affect function of the left kidney. The mechanism for this relationship is obscure, but may involve the circulatory system in some way. Specifically, a decrease in the motility of the left kidney is often seen in patients with sexual dysfunction. Function of the left kidney also has a significant emotional component. Whenever there is a strong emotional or psychological shock, the motility of the left kidney decreases.

Renal problems may be associated with venous problems of the left testicle or left labium majus. The left ovarian (or testicular) vein opens into the left renal vein, whereas its counterpart on the right opens directly into the inferior vena cava *(Illustration 9-4)*. A renal ptosis on the left side (but not the right) can therefore put this vein at an abnormal angle with the renal vein, leading to restricted venous return accompanied by functional problems. For example, we have observed that it is more common for the cervix to be restricted on the left, and believe that this is related to the venous asymmetry. Other related problems (e.g., discomfort and localized pain) increase in women during the premenstrual period, and in men after sexual activity or defecation.

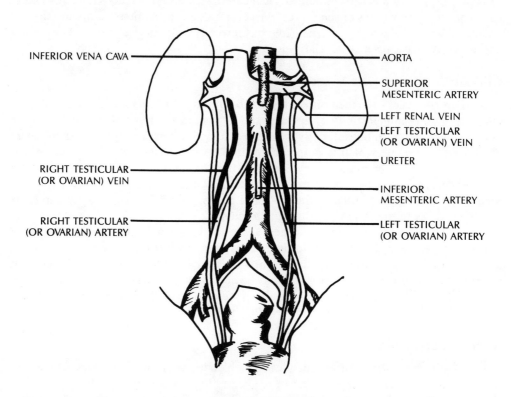

Illustration 9-4
Venous Return from the Genitals

We treated two cases of left-sided testicular varicose veins in which the simple act of mobilizing the kidney upward reduced the congestion and discoloration immediately (albeit temporarily). When the varicosities are not too severe, manipulation can have a curative effect.

Similarly, there are reflux phenomena involving movement of blood between the ovarian (or testicular) vein and left renal vein, due to changes in venous pressure in this area during sexual activity. These are not caused by problems with renal mechanics, but the symptoms are similar.

Symptoms

Renal ptosis can present a variety of signs and symptoms. Some are nonspecific. For example, the patient has difficulty holding the arms up for more than a brief period because of the stretching of the fascial system, which affects the kidneys. As always, you should be observant. The patient characteristically is forward bent and holds his stomach and/or the lower ribs. When he coughs or sneezes, he flexes the ipsilateral thigh to counteract the increase in pressure.

When the kidney moves downward, it brings along only the proximal part of the ureter (which arises from the medial edge of the kidney). The rest of the ureter remains fixed to the parietal peritoneum by fibrous tissue. The elbow which is thus formed has an influence on urinary excretion and fluid dynamics. This resistance to flow may favor the development of kidney stones. In this situation, the longitudinal tension of the ureter is reduced, compromising its smooth muscle tone. Also, traction exerted on the peritoneum by the ptosed kidney contributes to the production of spasms of the intestine. This abnormally increased intestinal tonus can compress the ureter and also reverse urinary flow. In some instances, this will result in low back pain.

Many other signs have been mentioned already, but I would like to summarize selected ones here, with a few additions:

- sensation of discomfort and weight in the lower abdomen, often worsened by inhalation or other abdominal efforts
- the intestinal phase of digestion is laborious and prolonged due to spasms caused by the kidney, producing a slight sick feeling which is aggravated by foods that place special demands on the intestines (cabbage, cucumbers, fatty foods, etc.)
- deep abdominal discomfort about fifteen minutes after fluid intake, particularly if the patient drinks too much and too quickly
- narrow belts (which aggravate the mechanical restrictions) are poorly tolerated, whereas the patient may selectively prefer wide belts, especially with second degree ptosis
- accentuation of problems at the end of the day or after prolonged labor
- low back pain following a characteristic pattern: it is felt upon awakening, and improves within 10-30 minutes after standing up. In the late afternoon the pain returns and progresses until it is difficult to tolerate by evening. Within 10 minutes after going to bed the pain disappears. The pain on awakening can be explained by nervous irritation, vascular and peritoneal spasms, and renal congestion during the night
- slight thigh and knee discomfort (more of a hypersensitivity or numbness than a true pain), increasing during the day
- sciatica originating from chronic contractions of the lumbar musculature, in combination with other factors. Sciatica secondary to renal problems is rarer on the left than the right
- systolic arterial pressure is often lower on the side of the ptosed kidney, even if the patient is hypertensive. When you find an elevated systolic pressure in a hypertensive patient, freeing the kidney can sometimes decrease this pressure.

From an energetic viewpoint, the kidney is responsible for the deep layers of the body's energies. It has a strong relationship to the liver; so strong, in fact, that liver dysfunction is generally an indication for treatment of the kidneys, and vice versa.

OTHER DISORDERS

Although ptoses are common and worthy of attention, we must remember that many other diseases of the kidney do exist. In this section, I will briefly describe a number of less-common renal disorders which present a variety of symptoms and etiologies.

Renal Insufficiency

ACUTE: Acute renal insufficiency applies to cases of markedly decreased urinary output secondary to injury of the renal parenchyma. Renal blood flow can fall by as much as half its normal value. Possible causes include:

- tubular necrosis following a trauma or severe illness, in association with shock or intense renal vasoconstriction, all of which lead to decreased perfusion of the kidneys
- hemolysis and hypotension following surgical intervention
- injury with severe muscle damage leading to large release of myoglobin (which is nephrotoxic), plus vasoconstriction and shock
- childbirth
- formation of casts which block the tubular lumens.

Clinical symptoms include anuria (no urination) or oliguria (scanty urination), murky or blood-stained urine, nausea, prolonged drowsiness, muscular weakness, thirst, cardiovascular or pulmonary complications, septicemia (usually from *Staphylococcus*), anemia, and convulsions.

Differential diagnosis should consider obstruction of the ureters or bladder (which can also prevent urine formation), malignant growths, and idiopathic fibrosis around the ureters.

CHRONIC: This condition involves a reduction in functional renal tissue. There are fewer active nephrons, and these tend to undergo hypertrophy. Symptoms include increased urea excretion and initial polyuria (excessive urine production), diminishing gradually as renal insufficiency sets in. The patient drinks and excretes more water in order to eliminate the normal quantities of solutes, resulting in polyuria, polydipsia (excessive thirst), and nocturia (excessive urination at night). The latter phenomenon provokes sensations of intense thirst or hunger before or upon awakening, which can then turn into nausea and vomiting. To prevent this, advise the patient to drink after nocturnal urination.

Because of urinary excretion, vomiting, and diarrhea, the patient tends to lose sodium, resulting in signs such as dry mouth, loss of normal skin tone, tiredness, nausea, fainting, cramps, muscular fibrillation, and occasionally convulsions.

Other clinical symptoms of chronic renal insufficiency can be listed as follows:

- weakness, tiredness, insomnia, dyspnea, anorexia, headache
- persistent nausea, bad taste in the mouth, pallor, drowsiness, hiccoughs
- itching of the limbs, retinopathy
- hypertension, pulmonary edema
- digestive symptoms (inflammation of the parotid gland, ulcers of the buccal mucosa due to the presence of urea in the saliva, acidosis, dehydration)

- neuromuscular signs (nocturnal muscular cramps from lack of calcium)
- hematological signs (anemia resulting from hemolysis and reduced bone marrow function)
- cutaneous signs (olive-colored skin due to accumulation of pigments similar to carotene, dry skin, calcium deposits, itching)
- infectious complications.

Glomerulonephritis

ACUTE: Glomerulonephritis is an inflammation of the kidneys in which the glomeruli are primarily affected. The acute form usually follows by 1-3 weeks a group A beta-hemolytic streptococcal infection. It may also follow other bacterial, viral, or parasitic infections such as bacterial endocarditis, sepsis, hepatitis, typhoid fever, mumps, measles, or mononucleosis. In the latter cases, the problem is usually milder than in the post-streptococcal variety. With this disorder, the kidneys are of a normal or increased size, their surface is dotted with small hemorrhages, and the renal pyramids are congested. After recovery, the kidneys may be fibrosed and atrophied. Clinical symptoms include:

- chest pain
- fever (minimum 38.5 °C)
- initial malaise followed by general fatigue and anorexia
- scanty and dark urine
- swelling of the ankles and eyelids
- dyspnea, abdominal pain, nausea
- hypertension, headache, possible convulsions.

CHRONIC: Chronic glomerulonephritis is actually a collection of disorders which affect the glomerular capillaries and provoke cicatricial (scarring) modifications. The disease is more frequent in men under 40 years of age, and follows acute glomerulonephritis or simple infection. It can be present without symptoms for as long as 10 years. Possible symptoms include general fatigue, anemia, dyspnea, hypertension, oliguria, presence of proteins and red blood cells in the urine, normal-sized kidneys, renal insufficiency, and pulmonary edema.

Chronic Pyelonephritis

This chronic form of nephritis, affecting primarily the interstitial tissue, seems to result from recurrent bacterial infections. While some patients have anatomical urinary tract abnormalities (e.g., obstruction, or reflux from the bladder into the ureters), the urinary tract usually appears normal. The urine in the bladder is usually sterile, but when it is not, bacteria are able to travel from the bladder to the kidney via the column of urine which connects these two organs.

This disorder originates from pyelitis (inflammation of the renal pelvis) in children, a urinary infection during pregnancy or, more rarely, an acute form of pyelonephritis. It may progress very slowly. Symptoms, which are highly variable and sometimes absent, include episodes of unexplained fever accompanied by low back pain, cloudy urine, albumin in the urine, general fatigue and listlessness, anorexia, and hypertension. The kidneys are often fibrous and of differing sizes.

Kidney Stones

Kidney stones (or renal lithiasis) are manifested by extremely painful attacks which originate in the flank or back and radiate to the lower abdomen, genital organs, and/or medial thighs. Sometimes the pain resembles that of biliary colic, appendicitis, gastroduodenal ulcer, or low back pain. Chronic dehydration and sedentary lifestyle are frequent causes. Hyperparathyroidism, excessive milk intake, or highly alkaline diet (all tending to produce hypercalciuria, or excessive calcium in the urine) can also be involved. Less common symptoms are pain on urination, and presence of blood or albumin in the urine.

LOW BACK PAIN

This is certainly the most common presenting symptom in our practice. The more patients we treat, the more we realize that low back pain hides a multitude of dysfunctions. We have seen at least twenty cases of low back pain due to renal problems in young people. In a typical case, the patient first reported chest pain which resolved with standard antibiotic therapy. Several weeks later, low back pain appeared, along with pain in the lower limbs (particularly the knees). Scanning, IVP, and biochemical examinations were negative. The patient was tired and arterial pressure was slightly elevated. Examination showed that the kidneys had lost their motility. Manipulation of the lumbar spine gave no results, but the problem resolved following visceral manipulation.

For these cases, spinal manipulation is not only not helpful, but can exacerbate the problem by further irritating the affected structures. Induction of the kidneys and liver is sometimes helpful (we often send these patients to see a homeopath or acupuncturist). As mentioned, pyelonephritis or glomerulonephritis can evolve very gradually over a long period, with no symptoms for several years.

In female patients who seek treatment for low back pain, the actual problem sometimes turns out to be reflux from the bladder into the ureters. With children, low back pain should never be viewed as primarily a musculoskeletal disorder. It is almost always the reflection of a visceral pathology. If the child is chronically fatigued, listless, tires easily, or is a late developer, the problem could be chronic pyelonephritis.

ASSOCIATED PATHOLOGIES AND SYMPTOMS

Besides the primary renal disorders discussed above, I would like to mention a few related pathological considerations, and give an overview of symptoms which are of interest in the context of visceral manipulation.

Abnormalities of the renal pelvis in a overly mobile kidney provoke hydronephrosis because of a partial (and sometimes intermittent) obstruction of the ureter. Thus, ptosis of a mobile kidney inevitably brings about problems of urinary circulation. The pain of hydronephrosis is aggravated by exercise and increased fluid intake, and is alleviated by the supine position. Interestingly, the same is true of a ptosis.

Among the symptoms of a polycystic kidney is posteroinferior abdominal pain, caused by the weight of the kidney pulling on its vascular and nervous attachments and on adjacent structures. This pain increases with exercise and decreases with rest. Again, these signs remind us of a ptosis. Do not hesitate to send your patient for outside consultation if you are less than totally confident in your diagnosis.

Following are some common symptoms which often reflect minor renal dysfunction and respond well to visceral manipulation. Always check renal mobility and motility if any of these signs are present:

- intense early morning or late night thirst, sometimes enough to wake the patient
- hunger on arising, sometimes giving way to nausea or malaise
- low back pain on awakening, improving soon after standing up
- exaggerated reflexes, muscular weakness, intermittent tetany
- darkened or cloudy urine
- intense itching, particularly of the lower limbs
- gingivitis, chronic aphthous ulcers, minor infections of the oral cavity
- fatigue or lethargy
- indigestion with slow transit
- variations in blood pressure
- low back and abdominal discomfort during the day
- flaky, dehydrated skin.

Diagnosis

As usual, simple observation can provide significant diagnostic clues. A patient with renal restrictions will tend to forward bend and sidebend toward the side of the restriction. With one hand, he holds the posterolateral trunk or lower abdomen. He is uncomfortable standing still. The legs are taut and he often flexes the ipsilateral thigh.

PALPATION

Palpation of a kidney is not easy. As mentioned at the beginning of the chapter, students and inexperienced practitioners often believe they are touching the inferior pole of a kidney when they are actually collecting and shaping a portion of the intestinal mass, or feeling the bend between the descending and inferior duodenum. Fortunately for our purposes, a ptosed kidney is easier to reach than a non-ptosed one because it has moved anteriorly. Your approach should be gentle to avoid creating intestinal contractions which could disrupt your techniques and cause discomfort for the patient.

To palpate the right kidney, with the patient in the supine position, place yourself on his right and look for the ascending colon. Surround it with your thumbs on its lateral edge and with your fingers on its medial edge. Next, move medially by placing both thumbs on the medial edge of the ascending colon and the fingers on the lateral edge of the descending duodenum *(Illustration 9-5)*. If you are successful, the kidney will be felt deeply between the thumbs and fingers. Place the hypothenar eminence in the gap between the duodenum and colon, and push it in deeply. If the kidney is in a normal position, you should be able to feel its anterior surface (which is smooth and bulging), without feeling the inferior edge. The impression is like feeling a bar of soap.

If the kidney is ptosed, you will be able to reach the inferior pole by moving your pressure inferiorly. With a second degree ptosis, you will feel more of the anteromedial part of the kidney, because of its external rotation. With a very slender patient with poor muscle tone, you may be able to feel the inferior edge. On palpation of a third degree

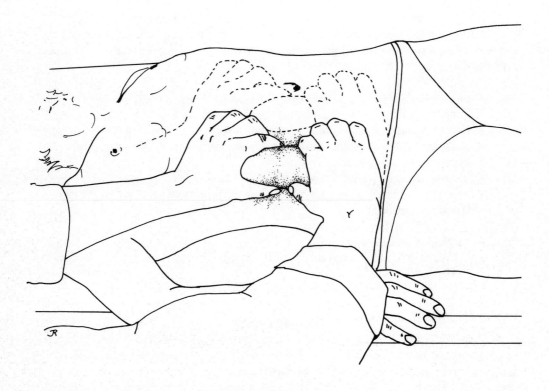

Illustration 9-5
Palpation of the Right Kidney

ptosis, instead of having the inferior edge under the heel of your hand, you will feel the upper part or even the superior edge, and the kidney will feel extremely mobile. Any time you find the inferior edge of the kidney under the line connecting the two ASIS's, the kidney will be easy to palpate because it is so superficial.

The left kidney is found about 1.5 cm higher than the right. To palpate it, start by finding the surface projection of the duodenojejunal flexure, which is symmetrically opposite that of the sphincter of Oddi. This flexure is a fixed point often used as a landmark in radiology. It is deep to the peritoneum, omentum, small intestine, and stomach, and appears as a round mass about the size of a quarter. Place the thenar or hypothenar eminence just inferior to this point and push it posteriorly as far as possible. Move your pressure inferiorly and you will feel the anterior left renal mass.

LISTENING

On general listening, the patient first sidebends toward the side of the restricted kidney and, only afterward, rotates toward that side and forward bends. The degree of forward bending is usually related to the degree of ptosis. Unfortunately, the kidney is a retroperitoneal organ and it is difficult to obtain precise diagnostic information by general listening.

Local listening enables you to differentiate the degree of ptosis, primarily by focusing on whether there is internal or external rotation. Place your hand over the surface projection of the kidney (usually with the heel of the hand at the level of the umbilicus). Press the hand slightly posteriorly and then concentrate on attracting the tissues into your palm (inhalation aids in this process). Absence of motion usually indicates that the kidney is either restricted or fixed, but can be normal. This "frozen" state is common in first degree ptoses. External rotation of your hand indicates second degree ptosis. Internal rotation is most commonly due to third degree ptosis, but can also result from problems of the renal pelvis (e.g., kidney stones).

Listening to the motility of the kidney is accomplished by using less pressure, but extending the sense of touch through your hands. It permits you to differentiate between a "frozen" kidney and a normal kidney without restriction; in either case, there is no motion on local listening. A kidney without restriction will have normal motility, with good expir and inspir. A frozen kidney will not only have no motion on local listening, it will also have no motility. Our experience suggests that utilization of both local listening and listening for motility is essential for satisfactory diagnosis and formulation of treatment. Palpation for mobility alone cannot correctly evaluate the rotation of the kidney.

DIFFERENTIAL DIAGNOSIS

With the patient in the supine position, legs bent, place the heel of your hand just above the umbilicus, middle finger on the midline (Illustration 9-6). With a renal problem (arrow 1), the palm is pulled deeply posteriorly, then laterally to the right or left (depending on the affected kidney), and finally slightly superomedially. In the presence of renal ptosis, the palm moves initially away from the midline, then inferolaterally for a second degree, or inferomedially for a third degree ptosis. This is the best diagnostic means of differentiating the degree of ptosis.

For the sphincter of Oddi, the thenar eminence carries out a pronation rather than a transverse movement, moves obliquely upward on the right midclavicular-umbilical line, and stops two or three fingers' width above the umbilicus. For the descending duodenum, the thenar eminence turns onto its radial edge, the thumb resting 2 cm to the right of the umbilicus, on a line parallel to the midline. For the pylorus, the palm, which is attracted upward, situates itself two or three fingers' width below the xiphoid process, to the left or the right depending on the position of the pylorus.

For the right ureter, the hand turns onto its radial edge slightly to the right of the umbilicus, and moves inferiorly. In the case of a calculus, the radial edge of the thenar eminence moves posteriorly with a slight clockwise rotation. We suggest that you practice locating calculi which have already been found independently by scanning or IVP. For the cecum, the palm moves inferiorly and to the right.

The duodenojejunal flexure presents the most difficult differential diagnosis (arrow 2) because it is located directly in front of the left kidney and is often in spasm. For a dysfunction of this flexure, the hypothenar eminence slides superiorly and to the left. The palm pushes in with a slight clockwise rotation, whereas for the kidney it moves more posteriorly and then superiorly. For the gastric fundus (arrow 3), the hand leaves the umbilical region and moves superiorly and to the left, toward the costal margin. For the pancreas, the middle finger leaves the midline and moves superiorly and to the left, creating a 30° angle with a transverse plane passing slightly superior to the umbilicus.

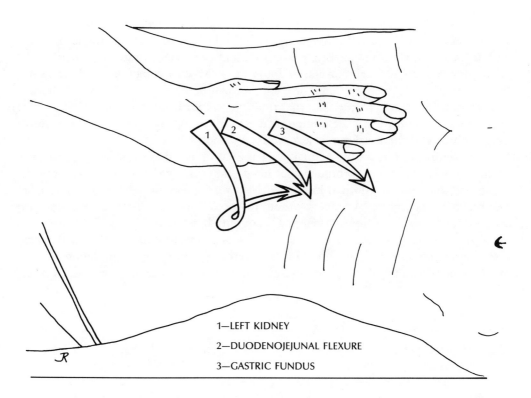

1—LEFT KIDNEY
2—DUODENOJEJUNAL FLEXURE
3—GASTRIC FUNDUS

Illustration 9-6
Local Differential Diagnosis: Left Side

DIAGNOSTIC MANIPULATION

As shown previously for other organs, manipulation can be used to clarify the diagnosis. The aggravation technique for the right kidney is performed with the patient in the seated position and slightly kyphosed. Place your fingers on the right costal margin, flat under the liver and as far posteriorly as possible, and push the abdominal mass inferiorly. In the case of a ptosis the patient will feel discomfort or posterior costal pain, sometimes with radiation toward the lower abdomen.

The corresponding relief technique consists of bringing the liver posterosuperiorly. However, this technique will be useless with a third degree ptosis because the loss of any renal connection with the liver and diaphragm prevents the lifting from having any effect.

Costal pressure can also be used as an aggravation technique. The patient sits with his hands behind the neck. With one hand, lift the elbows to put him into straight backward bending and, with the other, apply direct anterior pressure on the posterior angle of R11. With a renal problem, the patient feels discomfort or lumbar pain and holds his breath. However, a mechanical costovertebral restriction can give the same result.

You need to know if you are dealing with an injury to the actual renal parenchyma or the renal attachments. Palpation of a kidney can be sensitive, or even slightly uncomfortable, but should not be painful or produce a protective reflex. If it does, you are using too much force. Perform a recoil technique by pushing the inferior pole of the kidney superiorly along the longitudinal renal axis as far as you can, and then release it quickly. Sensitivity to this technique indicates a problem with the ligamentary renal attachments.

ASSOCIATED SKELETAL RESTRICTIONS

With first and second degree ptoses, there are restrictions at the level of T7 and T11 and their ribs. In third degree ptosis, there is no connection with the diaphragm and therefore no thoracic restrictions. With the first and second degrees, there may be restrictions of L1-L4 resulting from irritation of the psoas muscle and the iliohypogastric, ilioinguinal (both L1), genitofemoral (L1-L2), lateral femoral cutaneous (L2-L3), and femoral (L2-L4) nerves, plus the effects of peritoneal and spinal nerve root stretching.

There may be involvement of the knee because of its innervation by the femoral nerve, and the navicular, first cuneiform and fifth metatarsal bones because they are reflexogenic (i.e., trigger points). The lower limbs may also be involved in kidney disorders secondary to poor biomechanics or problems caused by contractions of the psoas muscle.

We have found it extremely helpful to work on the lower limbs every time we work on a kidney (or the cecum or sigmoid colon). Otherwise, the effect of treatment will be more temporary. Try putting one hand on the superior surface of the foot and perform local listening, following the palm until it comes to rest. If it moves, it usually goes toward either the tibia or fibula. Check to see if this restriction is related to a kidney problem, using the other hand to inhibit the kidney by pushing up on it slightly. If the leg restriction disappears, it is secondary to a kidney problem; if there is no change, it is a local phenomenon.

One may find glenohumeral periarthritis of renal origin. On the right, this is more likely to be associated with abnormal tension of the fascial system or, on the left, of reflex origin. Perform the glenohumeral articulation test (see chapter 1) with one hand, and with the other perform a relief technique or utilize an inhibition point. Improvement of mobility confirms renal participation.

BLOOD PRESSURE

In general, with mechanical renal injury, ipsilateral arterial pressure decreases. Confusingly, blood pressure tends to increase with problems of the parenchyma, but the side of the mechanically affected kidney will still have a relatively lower pressure. An additional complication occurs with hydronephrosis, where the kidney is ptosed but arterial pressure is raised.

The Adson-Wright test is often positive on the affected side with first and second degree ptosis. This test can be used to confirm renal disorders. It can also be performed before and after manipulation as a means of confirming your results.

DIGESTIVE SYMPTOMS

With kidney dysfunctions, adjacent portions of the intestine are affected directly by mechanical irritation, and also indirectly by reflex mechanisms. The patient feels discomfort during the intestinal phase of digestion, in the late afternoon, and around 1-2 A.M. A "pseudodigestive" sign is abdominal pain of renal origin which is exaggerated after drinking because the renal pelvises become distended.

Treatment

Our goal in treatment is not simply to "pull up" the kidney, i.e., change its position. As always in visceral manipulation, we wish to improve motility and mobility. In chapter 1, I described some dramatic increases in renal mobility achieved by Jacques-Marie Michallet with manipulation (see Appendix I). Nevertheless, we have altered the position of the kidney in some cases. Unfortunately, we cannot use ultrasound to document a ptosis, unless it is very severe. Another goal is to release any surrounding visceral restrictions or fibrotic attachments. By this means, vascular and urinary circulation are improved.

Before manipulating a restricted kidney, perform stretching techniques to release adhesions of the posterior lamina (part of the renal fascia) on the quadratus lumborum, or of the anterior lamina on the psoas muscle. This will save you a lot of time. Besides, these muscles are often in spasm due to mechanical irritation of their nerves.

RECOIL

Recoil techniques are used primarily to treat "frozen" kidneys, i.e., kidneys which seem to have no mobility and do not respond to the usual direct techniques *(Visceral Manipulation*, pp. 200-202). Try these techniques again after recoil has been applied 2-3 times. If there is still no improvement in mobility, the principal problem is not with the kidney.

The patient is supine, with his legs more or less bent depending on abdominal tension. Lengthening the psoas slightly can help make the kidney more anterior (and therefore easier to find), but may also make it less mobile. The inferior pole of the right kidney is usually around the level of the umbilicus between the ascending colon and duodenum; the left kidney is most easily found just posteroinferior to the duodenojejunal flexure.

For a ptosed kidney, touch the inferior pole with your hypothenar eminence and push it superomedially as far as possible. This technique is aimed not at repositioning the kidney, but at engaging its attachments and surrounding structures, and facilitating its motion. There are variations in the direction of the movement depending on the degree of ptosis being treated.

For first degree ptosis, recoil consists of pushing superomedially and slightly posteriorly as far as possible, and then quickly releasing your pressure. For second degree ptosis, the hand sidebends and externally rotates; recoil consists of pushing superomedially and (for the right kidney) from right to left in the same manner.

For third degree ptosis, successful manipulation is difficult. The kidney has descended to the point where it is no longer subject to the external rotation produced by the psoas. It rests on its medial edge, finds itself in internal rotation, and thus loses its oblique inferolateral direction. The latter phenomenon can be observed with IVP, where the vascular attachment of the kidney is less evident. The recoil technique for a third degree ptosis involves applying pressure from bottom to top, from medial to lateral, and from front to back. In case of difficulty, you can initially accentuate internal rotation by pushing in the direction of the lesion (this is true for any of these recoil techniques). However, too much force will create a restriction, and the resulting pain will prevent the necessary post-manipulative relaxation.

COMBINED DIRECT TECHNIQUE

The patient is in the supine position, with the leg on the affected side resting on your shoulder *(Illustration 9-7)*. For a second degree ptosis, mobilize the kidney by bringing it posterosuperiorly and medially. By moving your shoulder, you can adjust the tension of the psoas, thus varying the rotation of the kidney and how far it comes anteriorly. This combined technique enables us to utilize the "rail" of the psoas, and produce small isometric contractions of this muscle against resistance.

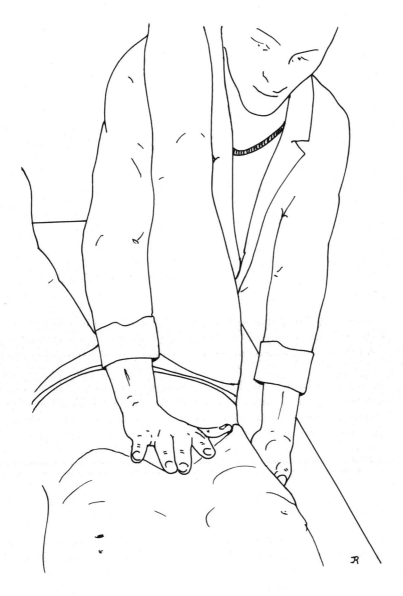

Illustration 9-7
Combined Direct Manipulation of the Kidney

With your free hand, hold the leg on the shoulder and ask the patient to lift it slightly. At the moment when contraction stops, mobilize the kidney, taking advantage of the relaxation which follows muscular activity.

GENERAL RELEASE TECHNIQUE

If you are unable to obtain results after several tries using the specific techniques described above, try the knee/elbow general release technique which we also use for the intestinal mass. The patient rests on his knees and forearms, thus bringing the abdomen anteriorly and slightly superiorly. You stand to the side and, reaching with one hand around the back, place the two hands so that the heels are just lateral to the edges of the rectus abdominis muscle on each side.

Bring your hands toward each other while pushing the abdominal mass posteriorly (i.e., toward the ceiling) in order to obtain a good hold. Keep your hands tightly together and stretch the abdominal contents anterosuperiorly. This will create deep abdominal traction which engages the posterior parietal peritoneum and retroperitoneal organs. The other directions that your hands take will depend on the restrictions in the abdomen. Repeat two or three times. This technique can be used with recoil.

POSTERIOR APPROACH

There is a weak lumbar point which makes it possible to approach the kidney posteriorly with minimal interference from intervening soft tissues; this is Grynfeltt's (or Lasshaft's) triangle, where aponeuroses of the internal and external abdominal oblique muscles are absent (Illustration 9-8). Place the patient in the supine or lateral decubitus position with legs bent. Place one or two fingers against the posterior aspect of R12 and move them simultaneously anteriorly and toward the iliac crest. When you meet a slight amount of resistance, mobilize the kidney anterosuperiorly, using the anterior hand to accentuate this movement. The inferior edge of the kidney is found on a horizontal plane going through the transverse process of L3. The fingers mobilize the kidney via the latissimus dorsi muscle, and the fibrous connective tissue layer representing the fused aponeuroses of the latissimus dorsi, internal and external oblique, and transversalis muscles. Against the posteroinferior portion of R12, three fingers' width from the spine, is the twelfth intercostal nerve; in the middle of Grynfeltt's triangle you can feel the ilioinguinal and iliohypogastric nerves.

This region is an efficient "trigger" zone, i.e., a very precise reflexogenic zone that can be used to start, accelerate and/or increase the effects of a treatment. For example, if you are working on the stomach with little or no effect, use this trigger zone on the left and things will start to happen (or happen more quickly).

Between R11/R12, the kidney is in direct contact with the pleural cul-de-sac, another trigger zone. To utilize this zone during treatment, apply pressure at three fingers' width from the spine, against the lateral border of the paravertebral muscles.

INTERACTION BETWEEN THE KIDNEYS

The two kidneys are connected by the renal fascia. Any factor restricting one will therefore affect the other. With right renal ptosis, the left kidney maintains a normal position. However, it does lose its motility, perhaps because of the abnormal tension exerted on the renal fascia. In third degree ptosis of the right kidney, this kidney becomes

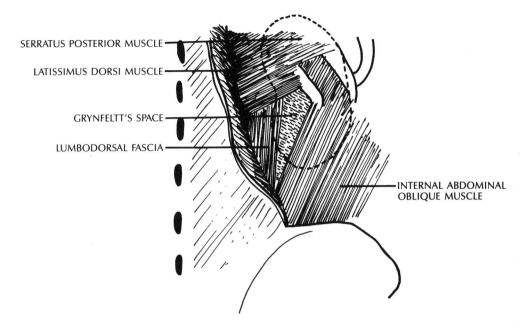

SERRATUS POSTERIOR MUSCLE

LATISSIMUS DORSI MUSCLE

GRYNFELTT'S SPACE

LUMBODORSAL FASCIA

INTERNAL ABDOMINAL
OBLIQUE MUSCLE

Illustration 9-8
Grynfeltt's Space (After Gregoire and Oberlin)

ectopic. Because there is no longer a "fascial brake" interconnecting the kidneys, motility of the left kidney is often preserved. As mentioned previously, a very ptosed kidney has less of a pathological effect on the body than one that is moderately ptosed.

URETERAL CALCULI

Many people who come to see us for low back pain turn out to be suffering from kidney stones. These are usually not large calculi, but tiny stones of which the patient is unaware. Nonetheless, they can cause significant pain in the lumbar area. With ureteral calculi (stones which lodge in the ureters), we can sometimes provide successful treatment, but not with serious attacks involving such extreme pain that it is not possible to get close enough to touch, much less treat, the patient. There are several narrow points in the ureter where stones may get caught (Illustration 9-9). These points are also reflexogenic.

On palpation, it is not possible to differentiate the ureter from surrounding structures. However, stones can often be detected with listening. Place the hand along the surface projection of the ureter, on a line going obliquely from the tenth and eleventh costochondral cartilages to a point two fingers' width lateral to the pubic symphysis (Illustration 9-10). Where there is a stone, the palm is strongly attracted posteriorly, and carries out a slight clockwise rotation. We have been able to verify this many times with stones previously documented by X-ray. A similar clockwise rotation occurs when there are cysts in the abdomen or pelvis.

Just below its origin, the ureter has a diameter of approximately 1 cm. At the "neck" of the ureter, 1.5 cm from its origin, its width decreases to 4 mm. This is where most

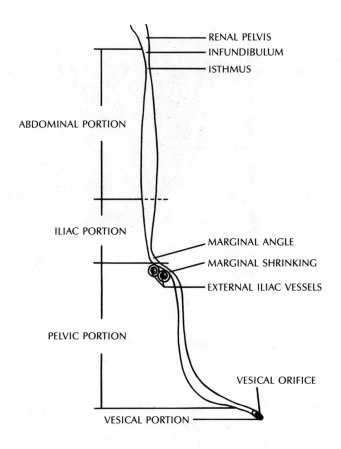

RENAL PELVIS
INFUNDIBULUM
ISTHMUS

ABDOMINAL PORTION

ILIAC PORTION

MARGINAL ANGLE
MARGINAL SHRINKING
EXTERNAL ILIAC VESSELS

PELVIC PORTION

VESICAL ORIFICE

VESICAL PORTION

Illustration 9-9
Narrow Points in the Ureter

stones are encountered. A second narrow point is found where the ureter crosses over the iliac vessels, on the line connecting the two ASIS's. The third narrowing is found at the junction of the ureter with the bladder, which can be directly manipulated via the vagina in women.

Ureteral calculi can be treated in two ways. In the direct technique, you start by marking the position of the stone, and then perform a compression/rotation at that point with the heel of the hand. At the end of the movement, push inferiorly to stretch the ureter, reinforcing its tone and peristaltic function.

In the indirect technique, the patient sits down with both hands crossed behind the neck. With one hand, hold both elbows; with the other, exert pressure just above the position of the stone. Bring the patient into backward bending, stretching the abdominal point downward.

TREATMENT STRATEGY

The right ("digestive") kidney is associated with the liver, descending duodenum, ascending colon, and cecum. The tension of these organs must be normalized prior to manipulation of this kidney. Pay particular attention to the cecum, which often has a causative role in renal ptosis. Test the posterior renal attachments and the ileocecal junction, which is often in spasm.

Before directly working on the left ("reproductive") kidney, free the duodenojejunal flexure, which is often taut and may produce restrictions of the kidney by reflex mechanisms. It is also a good idea to check the stomach attachments, and the motility of the ovaries.

Always finish manipulation with a combined technique on both kidneys at the same time, using direct manipulation followed by induction. In this, the hands perform a simultaneous movement in which the fingers join together superiorly, and the palms separate inferiorly. While testing and treating mobility in this way, pushing up on the

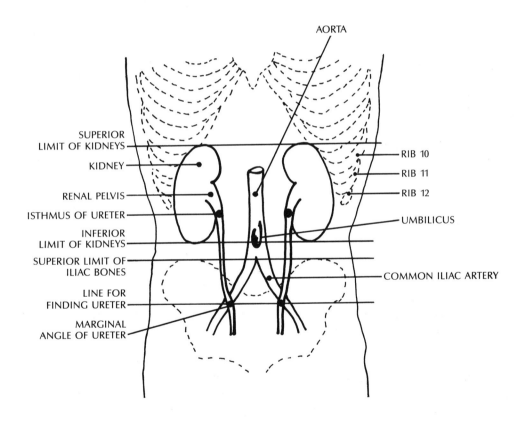

Illustration 9-10
Landmarks for Locating Renal Calculi

right kidney should result in transmitting a feeling of pressure to the left kidney, and vice versa. When doing induction, it is extremely important to leave the kidneys with good motion in both the expir and inspir phases, and to have the motions in sync. This combined technique has an overall stimulating effect on the patient.

Recommendations

With a ptosis, although the kidney is easy to palpate and the surrounding structures are sensitive, the kidney itself is rarely very painful. When a kidney is painful, consider hydronephrosis or a polycystic condition. Be very cautious with a kidney which is both sensitive (or painful), and also easy to palpate.

Never try to manipulate a kidney when there is fever or hematuria (blood in the urine). If the cause of the hematuria is known and not considered dangerous, you can work on the kidney after about a month; if the cause is unknown, refer the patient for a thorough clinical work-up.

Many digestive symptoms can actually reflect minor renal dysfunctions. A right renal ptosis, for example, gives numerous signs which could be incorrectly attributed to the cecum. Do not count on your patient's explanations for guidance.

Problems of the reproductive system often accompany a restriction of the left kidney, and vice versa. For example, there are many documented cases in which the presence of an intrauterine device affects the motility of the left kidney. With impotence problems in males, always test the motility of the left kidney.

Renal restrictions are often associated with costal restrictions, and almost always with problems of the coccyx. Consider treating a restricted rib before mobilizing the kidneys, especially in children, who are less likely to have primary restrictions of the kidney. Although we have not identified a definite link between the skull and the kidneys, we have observed in our practice that cranial restrictions presenting with concomitant kidney restrictions are usually posterior, and resolve quickly after treatment of the kidneys.

Always measure arterial pressure before and after renal manipulation. An inappropriate or poorly-executed technique may be revealed by a significant modification (i.e., imbalance between the two arms, hypotension, or hypertension), in which case you should consider alternative techniques.

ADVICE TO THE PATIENT

Urge a patient with a kidney problem to drink, but not in just any way he pleases. He should drink often, but in small amounts each time. Because it is difficult for people to change their habits, you should repeat this advice as often as necessary until it is consistently followed. Drinking too much at one time causes dilatation of the renal pelvis and ureters. This is often painful and makes the patient think that he is not "digesting" the water, so that he subsequently avoids drinking. In addition, the liquid should be warm. Warm water is assimilated easily, whereas cold water tends to "shock" the stomach, resulting in spasms or diminished peristaltic transit. Timing is also a factor; patients who ingest liquid two hours after a large meal, when intestinal activity is at its peak, will digest their food less well.

Closing Remarks

We have demonstrated in our practice that visceral manipulation is able to successfully relieve a multitude of structural and functional problems. Like all osteopathic methods, its success depends on the ability of our hands and mind. Our hands must be able to analyze the body's messages, and to sense and release abnormal tensions in the tissues.

As practitioners of this exacting discipline, we must have an understanding of the basic medical sciences, but it is the hands which distinguish the outstanding from the mediocre practitioner.

Appendix:
Kidney Mobilization and Ultrasound Documentation

Kidney Mobilization and Ultrasound Documentation

By Jacques-Marie Michallet[1]

Introduction

When the time came to choose a dissertation topic, my advisor, Jean-Pierre Barral, suggested that I do some research that would try to document in a scientific manner the results of an osteopathic technique. While the subjective improvement obtained by our treatments has been recognized by almost everyone, we are often criticized for failing to provide evidence that our actions have any objective effect.

M. Barral has been very interested in the kidneys for several years. During that time he has used such imaging techniques as fluoroscopy and intravenous pyelography (IVP) to demonstrate that when the kidneys develop ptosis or prolapse, there is a decrease in their mobility (i.e., their passive motion in response to breathing). He has also endeavored to show that this ptosis and decrease in mobility is often the source of such problems as recurrent urinary tract infections and renal lithiasis (due to dysfunctions in the flow of urine), and pain in the lower back and knees (due to irritation or compression of nerves). In addition, it is sometimes implicated in the development of hypertension and vascular problems of the kidneys themselves, or in venous flow upstream of the kidneys (such as those affecting the left testicular or ovarian veins).

M. Barral has shown that manipulation of the kidneys can relieve these problems, and has clearly demonstrated that the beneficial effects of manipulation are due to the return of normal kidney mobility, rather than the return to a normal anatomical position. This is because on follow-up radiographs, the kidneys have usually to some extent slipped back to the ptosed position. While it might be possible to use serial IVPs to demonstrate the effects of manipulation, there are a few major drawbacks to this method: they primarily

1. Thesis for the Diploma in Osteopathy at the European School of Osteopathy, Maidstone, Kent, United Kingdom, 1986. Edited and reprinted with the permission of the author.

measure position, which is not our goal; there is a risk of sensitivity to the contrast material, which can be life-threatening; and adequate testing before and after manipulation as well as on follow-ups would require too much radiation exposure for the subjects.

We therefore decided to use ultrasound, which does not present the risks of X-rays. The pictures obtained via ultrasound, however, appear as slices or sections of the body, and the kidneys cannot be located in relation to bony landmarks because such landmarks do not always appear in the section. To solve this problem, we then contacted a radiologist in Grenoble, Serge Cohen, M.D., whose competence and generosity had been utilized in M. Barral's earlier experiments. After due consideration, he suggested that it would be easy to measure the amount a kidney moved if we compared it to itself. When ultrasound is performed, two small crosses appear on the screen. These crosses are moveable. When they are aligned with two points on the screen, the machine automatically measures the distance between the two points, which is displayed on the screen in millimeters.

This enabled us to precisely measure kidney mobility by using the following method. One cross marker was aligned with a pole of the kidney at the end of inhalation. The other marker was aligned with the same pole at the end of exhalation. The machine then displayed the distance between these two points, which represented the mobility of that kidney. After making this measurement, we manipulated the kidney and then measured the mobility again in order to document the difference, if any.

On some of the photographs below, the small cross does not perfectly correspond to the edge of the renal pole. This is because there is a short interval between the time that one releases the handle to take the picture and when the picture is taken. Some patients were unable to hold their breath completely during this interval, which resulted in some movement. However, the measurements made by Dr. Cohen were correct and precise as he did align the crosses exactly with the edge of the renal pole before releasing the handle.

Anatomy and Physiology

Because this report is designed for practitioners who already have a good understanding of the anatomy and physiology of the kidney, I will only describe a few of the most important facts pertaining to kidney mobility.

- The kidney has no firm means of support (the pedicle of the kidney is incapable of serving this function). It has no suspensory ligament and no mesentery. The two main factors that prevent the kidney from falling down from its own weight are the "suction" of the thorax and the tension supplied by the anterior abdominal wall. The perirenal fat itself plays a supplementary role, as shown by the fact that when it is reduced suddenly it can be a factor in the development of renal ptosis.
- During inhalation the kidneys are pushed inferiorly along the "rail" of the psoas by the diaphragm. This gives them an oblique motion inferiorly and laterally with inhalation, and superiorly and medially with exhalation. The extent of this motion with deep inhalation and exhalation is between 5 cm and 10 cm, depending on the person.

In addition, when looking at a kidney ultrasound one can see that the superior pole is pushed forward by the diaphragm. Generally this motion is much less than the inferior and lateral motion, but it can be significant is some cases. We will see later that when this anterior rocking motion of the kidney is strong, it reduces the vertical amplitude of renal mobility.

- There are a multitude of factors that can reduce renal mobility. The most common are intervertebral (from T10 to L1) or costovertebral (R11 and R12) restrictions; gastric ptosis; inflammation or adhesion of a colic flexure; and renal ptosis, whether congenital (we will see such a case) or acquired (usually due to the sudden melting away of the perirenal adipose tissue, trauma, or childbirth). The degrees of renal ptosis and their pathophysiology have been fully discussed elsewhere (see *Visceral Manipulation*, p.199).

Experimental Protocol

We selected 25 people who, by our criteria, had markedly decreased mobility of one kidney. This diagnosis was reached by a variety of means: radiology (plain abdominal films or IVP); hypermobility of a kidney on osteopathic exam (primarily local listening); a history of recurrent urinary tract infection; or a history of sciatica or pain that radiated into the knee which did not seem to be due purely to musculoskeletal problems.

To make this study as objective as possible, and therefore to ensure that the measurements be as precise and reproducible as we could make them, it was necessary to define a protocol that would be adhered to in all cases. All right kidneys were measured at their superior pole in the supine position with the probe placed on the anterolateral aspect of the trunk. Left kidneys were measured at their inferior poles in the prone position with the probe placed in a posterolateral position. These positions were chosen after preliminary tests showed that other structures (primarily the cecum and colonic flexures) could otherwise interfere with the results.

In was also necessary to choose a single manipulative technique for the kidney and perform it in the same way in all cases. There are many techniques for manipulating the kidneys. The one we chose is performed with the subject seated, legs hanging unsupported, and hands resting on the knees. The practitioner stands behind the subject with his arms passed under the subject's arms. The subject's head and shoulders are forward bent in order to relax the abdominal wall, and the subject rotates slightly toward the side of the kidney to be manipulated. The practitioner slowly inches his fingers under the inferior pole of the kidney, and then pulls the kidney superiorly and slightly medially. The practitioner pulls while the subject exhales, and maintains this position during inhalation. This is repeated for four or five breathing cycles until a release is perceived. It is important both to be very gentle, so that the patient and the tissues are able to relax, and at the same time firm enough to have some effect.

After performing this technique, ultrasound was repeated in exactly the same manner as before. Two to four months later (depending on the subject's availability), we again repeated the ultrasound measurements. Each subject therefore underwent three measurements: before manipulation, immediately after manipulation, and a few months later.

Note that of the 25 cases described, we examined 24 right and one left kidney.

We believe that this overwhelming preponderance of right kidney problems is reflected in the daily clinical experiences of our colleagues. In any case, it is well known that the majority of ptosed and/or hypomobile kidney problems are found on the right. This is probably due to the mass of the liver weighing on the right kidney, as well as the fact that the right kidney is situated lower in the body than the left.

Cases

The presentation of each case includes the sex, age and pertinent information from the history and physical examination of the subject. We have also presented some examples of the ultrasounds themselves, and the results of treatment.

CASE 1: Mr. R. S., age 38. Thoracolumbar pain with a history of five small calculi seen on IVP a few years ago. The examination revealed a restriction of T12 (which we treated with manipulation) and hypomobility of the right kidney, which was slightly ptosed.

Initial measurement:	41 mm
Measurement after manipulation:	74 mm
Measurement 3 months later:	77 mm

Result: On his returns the patient reported that he no longer had back pain and had resumed athletic activities.

CASE 2: Mr. J. F., age 40. Recurrent thoracolumbar pain. With each acute episode there were restrictions at T11-L1. The history revealed that the episodes came after meals that were rich in meats and cheeses. On examination the right kidney was less mobile than the left.

Initial Measurement:	42 mm
Measurement after manipulation:	97 mm
Measurement 3 months later:	82 mm

Result: On his return, the patient reported no recurrence of pain.

CASE 3: Mrs. D. T., age 50. Recurrent cystitis and thoracolumbar pain. On examination the right kidney was in a slightly lowered position.

Initial Measurement:	74 mm
Measurement after manipulation:	86 mm
Measurement 4 months later:	87 mm

Result: On her return, the patient reported that she continued to have back pain, but no recurrence of cystitis. The gain in mobility was not very significant (12 mm), but the mobility was originally satisfactory and the improvement was sustained for four months.

CASE 4: Mr. J.R., age 53. Atypical thoracolumbar pain. Renal mobility seemed to be reduced on the right side.

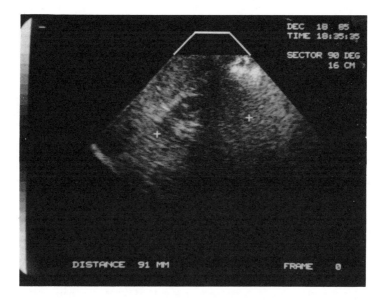

Initial measurement: 91 mm

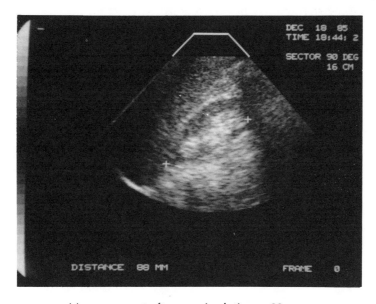

Measurement after manipulation: 88 mm

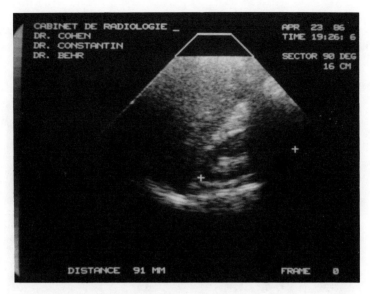

Measurement 4 months later: 91 mm

Result: This is a case of diagnostic error, as the original mobility was excellent. The reason for the small reduction in mobility (3 mm) is unclear, but was perhaps due to stress. In any event, it is comforting to see that four months later the mobility had returned to the original measurement, despite the efforts of the experimenter!

CASE 5: Mrs. M. L., age 58. Thoracolumbar pain with a history of frequent cystitis. On a previous IVP the right kidney had been ptosed.

Initial Measurement:	77 mm
Measurement after manipulation:	85 mm
Measurement 4 months later:	74 mm

Result: The mobility gained after manipulation was lost. The return visit of this patient occured shortly after she had been discharged from the hospital where she had been treated with steroids for a severe asthma attack. We speculate that this may have caused to a decrease in renal mobility.

CASE 6: Mrs. J.C., age 48. Thoracolumbar pain with a history of several attacks of renal colic and urinary tract infections. The right kidney seemed hypomobile.

Initial Measurement:	43 mm
Measurement after manipulation:	Approx. 56 mm
Measurement 4 months later:	61 mm

Results: Measurement immediately after manipulation was difficult due to intestinal gas. It is therefore unclear whether the relative increase between that measurement and four months later is real or artificial.

CASE 7: Ms. N. D., age 38. Atypical thoracolumbar pain with radiation into the knees. On examination the mobility of the kidneys was reduced, especially on the right.

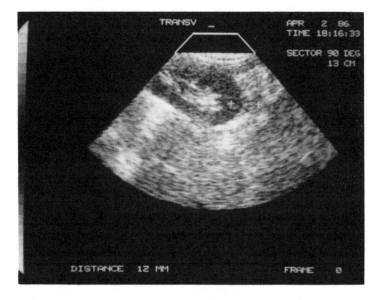

Initial measurement of right kidney: 12 mm

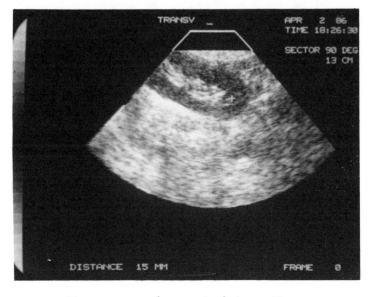

Measurement after manipulation: 15 mm

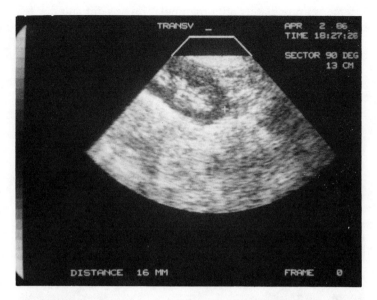

Measurement after manipulation of the left kidney: 16 mm

Results: We measured the mobility of the left kidney here because of the small amount of movement on the right, even after manipulation. Upon closer examination of the movement of these kidneys on the ultrasound screen, we discovered that this small vertical movement was replaced by a very large, anteriorly-directed rotational motion. Unfortunately, we were not able to precisely measure this rotational movement. The patient did return two months later, with no recurrence of back or knee pain.

CASE 8: Ms. M-O. M., age 34. Referred by our colleague, Didier Prat, with a diagnosis of right kidney hypomobility, and very frequent cystitis.

Initial Measurement:	57 mm
Measurement after manipulation:	62 mm
Measurement 4 months later:	59 mm

Results: As in case 7, analysis of the ultrasound screen showed a more significant rotational than vertical movement. On return, the patient stated that she had not had any attacks of cystitis since the last visit. This had not occurred for many years.

CASE 9: Ms. M-J. O., age 33. Referred by our colleagues, J.P. Barral and L. Rommeveaux, for attacks of renal colic and a ptosed right kidney.

Initial Measurement:	43 mm
Measurement after manipulation:	55 mm

Results: Unfortunately, it was not possible for this patient to return at a later date.

CASE 10 Ms. M.C., age 40. Referred by our colleagues, J.P. Barral and L. Rommeveaux, for lower back pain with a diagnosis of left kidney ptosis.

Initial Measurement (prone position):	76 mm
Initial Measurement (upright position):	76 mm
Measurement after manipulation:	104 mm

Results: In this patient the difference in mobility between the prone and upright positions was negligible. The patient was unable to return to the office, but she told us by phone that her back pain had disappeared.

CASE 11: Ms. A., age 44. Referred by our colleagues, J.P. Barral, for right-sided sciatica and knee pain with a diagnosis of right kidney hypomobility.

Initial Measurement:	44 mm
Measurement after manipulation:	47 mm
Measurement 5 months later:	59 mm

Results: The symptoms disappeared a few days after the mobilization of the kidneys, and have not reappeared. Note that there was a further gain in mobility of 12mm after five months.

CASE 12: Ms. N.V., age 49. History of lower back pain with radiation to the right sacroiliac joint and knee. On examination the right kidney felt hypomobile.

Initial Measurement:	38 mm
Measurement after manipulation:	56 mm
Measurement 4 months later:	62 mm

Results: There was both an increase in mobility and a disappearance of the symptoms.

CASE 13: Ms. J.A., age 44. History of atypical knee pain and frequent cystitis. On examination the right kidney felt hypomobile.

Initial Measurement:	58 mm
Measurement after manipulation:	95 mm
Measurement 2½ months later:	104 mm

Results: There was both an increase in mobility and a disappearance of the symptoms.

CASE 14: Mr. J-M. B., age 33. Recent episode of renal colic. Patient had had an IVP after his first episode of renal colic that showed a ptosed right kidney.

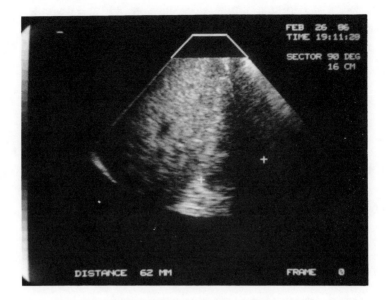

Initial measurement: 62 mm

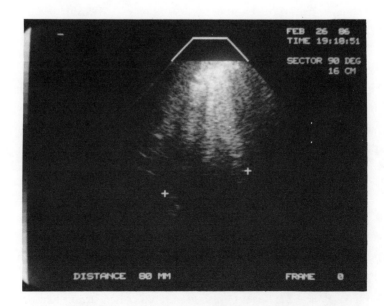

Measurement after manipulation: 80 mm

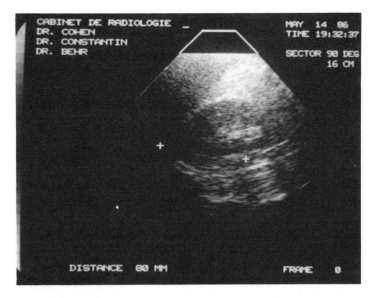

Measurement 2½ months later: 80 mm

Results: This patient had a short and wide body type, which we call brevilinear. This type of person has relatively less motion of his organs, so an increase in mobility of 18 mm was quite satisfactory.

CASE 15: Mr. C. A., age 47. History of a thoracolumbar pain which did not seem to be strictly due to musculoskeletal causes. On examination the right kidney felt hypomobile.

Initial Measurement:	60 mm
Measurement after manipulation:	63 mm
Measurement 3½ months later:	73 mm

Results: While the gain in mobility immediately brought about by manipulation was very small, the total increase was satisfactory.

CASE 16: Ms. B. B., age 28. History of frequent cystitis. An old IVP showed a ptosed right kidney.

Initial Measurement:	64 mm
Measurement after manipulation:	73 mm
Measurement 2 months later:	100 mm

Results: The increase in mobility that occured over two months was much greater than that from the initial response to manipulation. The symptoms of cystitis also disappeared.

CASE 17 Mr. C. B., age 29. Suffering from back pain. Old abdominal X-rays showed lithiasis of the right kidney.

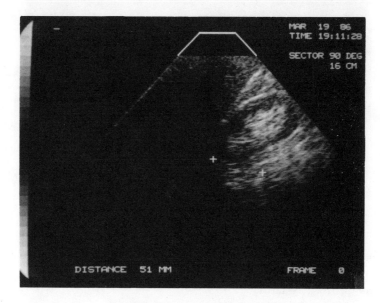

Initial measurement: 51 mm

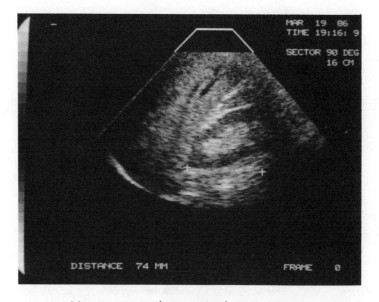

Measurement after manipulation: 74 mm

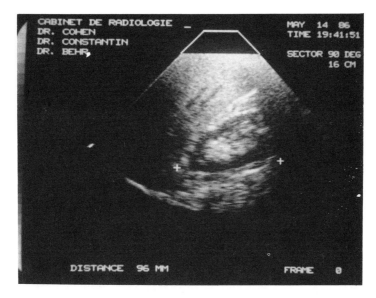

Measurement 2 months later: 96 mm

Results: The total increase in mobility was 45 mm, and the back pain disappeared.

CASE 18: Ms. C. C., age 47. Lower back pain and cystitis. An IVP taken a few years previously showed a ptosed right kidney and a significant bend in the right ureter.

Initial Measurement:	70 mm
Measurement after manipulation:	81 mm

Results: The patient was unable to return to the office for reexamination. She told us by telephone five months after the manipulation that she had no further symptoms of cystitis.

CASE 19: Ms. H. B., age not recorded. Referred by a colleague with a diagnosis of right kidney hypomobility.

Initial Measurement:	50 mm
Measurement after manipulation:	57 mm

Results: The patient was unable to return to the office for reexamination.

CASE 20: Ms. A. D., age 41. Recurrent cystitis that was particularly severe every spring. On examination the right kidney felt hypomobile.

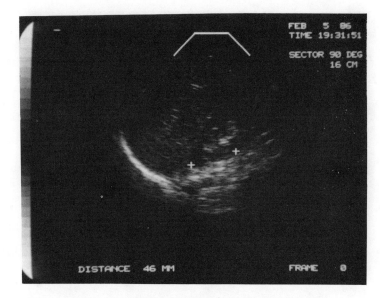

Initial measurement: 46 mm

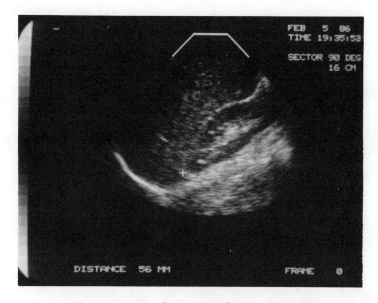

Measurement after manipulation: 56 mm

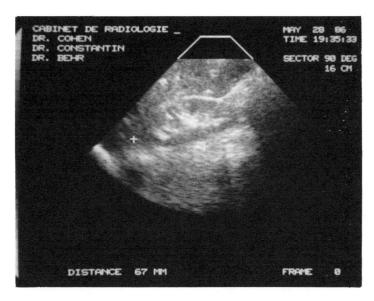

Measurement 3½ months later: 67 mm

Results: This patient was first seen in late winter. Since then she did not have any episodes of cystitis.

CASE 21: Mr. M. B., age 49. Atypical knee pain. On examination it was felt that the right kidney was hypomobile.

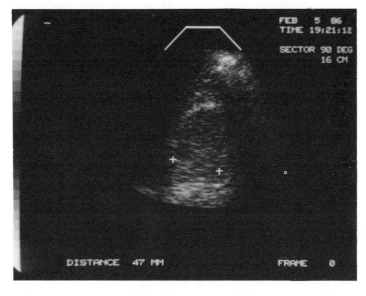

Initial measurement: 47 mm

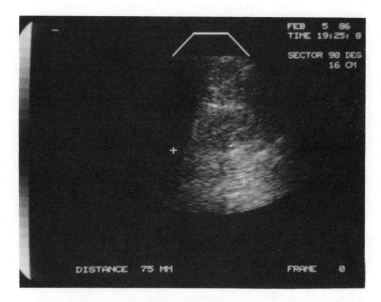

Measurement after manipulation: 75 mm

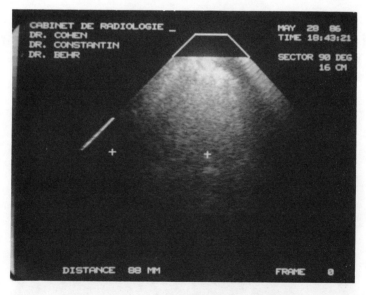

Measurement 3½ months later: 88 mm

Results: After treatment the knee pain disappeared and the patient was able to return to cycling, his favorite sport.

CASE 22 Ms. S. M., age 33. This patient came to be helped with infertility, but the history revealed that she suffered from frequent cystitis. On examination the right kidney felt hypomobile.

Initial Measurement:	27 mm
Measurement after manipulation:	64 mm
Measurement 3 months later:	69 mm

Results: During this period the patient had no episodes of cystitis.

CASE 23: Ms. M-L. A. P., age 59. Right flank pain with radiation into the right knee via the inguinal region.

Initial Measurement:	54 mm
Measurement after manipulation:	73 mm
Measurement 2 months later:	84 mm

Results: On reexamination the patient reported that the right flank and knee pain had disappeared, but that she still occasionally experienced pain in the inguinal region. We felt that this was due to a restriction of T12 and corrected it.

CASE 24: Ms. S. M., age 49. Hypetension with blood pressure of 180/100 mmHg, despite taking an antihypertensive diuretic. On examination the right kidney felt hypomobile.

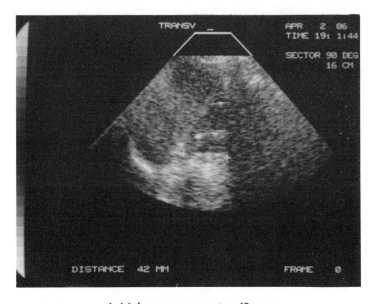

Initial measurement: 42 mm

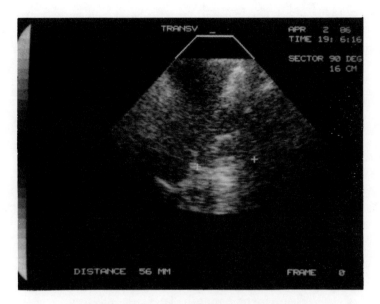

Measurement after manipulation: 56 mm

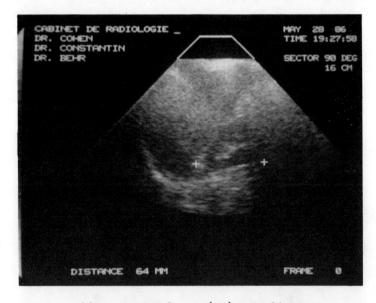

Measurement 2 months later: 64 mm

Results: The patient stopped taking the diuretic the day of the manipulation. On reexamination she reported that her blood pressure had never risen above 140/90 mmHg during the previous two months.

CASE 25: Ms. B. L., age not recorded. Referred by our colleague, Louis Rommeveaux, for verification of a right ectopic kidney, visible by IVP in the right iliac fossa.

Results: On ultrasound the right kidney was completely immobile while the left kidney had compensated by becoming hypertrophic. This is probably a congenital anomaly. No photo of the ultrasound was taken.

Conclusion

Of the cases studied, only two did not manifest a clear and easily measured increase in mobility after manipulation. One of these (case 4) was included in the study by diagnostic error because its mobility was originally well within the range of normal. In the other case (case 25) the kidney was totally fixed and in the iliac fossa so that it could not be reached. This supports our contention that visceral mobility is not only a real phenomena, but one that can be positively influenced by manipulation.

There was definitely variation in the amplitude of mobility. In general, the smallest amplitudes were found among subjects with the smallest stature, while taller subjects had larger amplitudes. This is logical. The average gain in amplitude after manipulation was 17.2 mm (eliminating the cases 4 and 25), with the extremes being 3 mm and 55 mm.

Another important aspect of this study was to measure the lasting effects of renal manipulation, that is, the extent to which the increase in amplitude remained when the subject was reexamined. Of the 23 cases, we were unable to reexamine four and in one other (case 5) the results were probably altered by treatment with large dosages of steroids. Of the remaining 18 cases in which we were able to do a follow-up examination 2-6 months after manipulation, 16 cases showed a further increase in renal mobility, a so-called "delayed reaction." In case 14 the mobility remained unchanged, and in case 2 there was a decrease in 15 mm of the post-treatment mobility, but still an increase of 40 mm in comparison to the pretreatment mobility. The average increase in mobility of these 18 cases at reexamination versus the original measurements was 25.8 mm, that is, 8.6 mm more than the immediate increase in mobility after manipulation. Why does this happen? We believe this is closely related to an adage attributed to the father of osteopathy, A.T. Still: "Find it, fix it, and leave it alone." This means that when we find a lesion or restriction we must treat it *a minima* and let nature do the rest. Once we have given the body the right stimulus, it does the rest on its own. This hypothesis is integral to the framework of osteopathic philosophy.

Acknowledgements

I would like to thank all of our teachers, particularly those who made this study possible, namely Jean-Pierre Barral, Serge Cohen, and Francois Dupont. I would also like to thank my senior colleagues who lavished advice and encouragement on me and my classmates, without whom I may have failed.

From the bottom of my heart I thank my relatives and friends for all their patience and affection during this project, when I badly neglected them.

Finally, I would like to dedicate this work to Louis Michallet, my father, who was a doctor in the noblest sense of the term. I unhappily lost him before I was able to speak to him in a meaningful way about osteopathic medicine. This will always remain the greatest regret in my life.

Bibliography

Barral, J-P.; Mathieu, J-P.; Mercier, P. *Diagnostic articulaire vertébral*. Charleroi: S.B.O.R.T.M., 1981.

Barral, J-P.; Mercier, P. *Visceral Manipulation*. Seattle: Eastland Press, 1988.

Bochuberg, C. *Traitement ostéopathique des rhinites et sinusites chroniques*. Paris: Maloine, 1986.

Braunwald, E. et. al., eds. *Harrison's Principles of Internal Medicine*. NY: McGraw-Hill, 1987.

Chauffour; Guillot. *Le Lien mécanique ostéopathique*. Paris: Maloine, 1985.

Contamin, R.; Bernard, P.; Ferrieux, J. *Gynécologie générale*. Paris: Vigot, 1977.

Cruveilhier, J. *Traité d'anatomie humaine*. Paris: Octave Doin, 1852.

Davenport, H.W. *Physiologie de l'appareil digestif, 2nd ed*. Paris: Masson, 1976.

Delmas, A. *Voies et centres nerveux, 10th ed*. Paris: Masson, 1975.

Dousset, H. *L'Examen du malade en clientèle, 6th ed*. Paris: Maloine, 1972.

Grégoire, R.; Oberlin, S. *Précis d'anatomie*. Paris: J.P. Baillère, 1973.

Herman, J.; Cier, J.F. *Précis de physiologie*. Paris: Masson, 1977.

Issartel, L.&M. *L'Ostéopathie exactement*. Paris: Robert Laffont, 1983.

Kahle, W.; Leonhardt, H.; Platzer, W. *Anatomie des viscères.* Paris: Flammarion, 1978.

Kamina, P. *Anatomie gynécologique obstétricale.* Paris: Maloine, 1984.

Korr, I. *The Neurobiologic Mechanisms in Manipulative Theory.* NY: Plenum, 1978.

Laborit, H. *L'Inhibition de l'action. biologie, physiologie, psychologie, sociologie.* Paris: Masson, 1981.

Lansac, J.; Lecomte, P. *Gynécologie pour le practicien.* Villeurbanne: S.I.M.E.P., 1981.

Malinas, Y.; Favier, M. *Gynécologie-Obstétrique.* Paris, Masson, 1979.

Renaud, R.; Sermet, J.; Ritter, J.; Bohler, J.L.; Eberst, B.; Gamerre, M.; Jacquemin, B.; Serment, G. *Les Incontinences urinaires chez la femme.* Paris: Masson, 1982.

Robert, J.G.; Palmer, R.; Boury-Heyler, C.; Cohen, J. *Précis de gynécologie.* Paris: Masson, 1974.

Rouvier, H. *Anatomie humaine.* Paris: Masson, 1967.

Scali, P.; Warrell, D.W. *Les Prolapsus vaginaux et l'incontinence urinaire chez la femme.* Paris: Masson, 1980.

Taurelle, R. *Obstétrique.* Paris: France Médical Edition, 1980.

Testut, L. *Traité d'anatomie humaine.* Paris: Octave Doin, 1889.

Testut, L.; Jacob, O. *Anatomie topographique.* Paris: Gaston Doin, 1922.

de Tourris, H.; Henrion, R.; Delecour, M. *Gynécologie et obstétrique.* Paris: Masson, 1979.

Upledger, J.E.; Vredevoogd, J.D. *Craniosacral Therapy.* Seattle: Eastland Press, 1983.

Waligora, H.; Perlemuter, L. *Anatomie.* Paris: Masson, 1975.

Williams, P.; Warwick, R., eds. *Gray's Anatomy.* Edinburgh: Livingstone, 1980.

Wright, S. *Physiologie appliquée à la médecine, 2nd ed.* Paris: Flammarion, 1974.

List of Illustrations

CHAPTER EIGHT

CHAPTER NINE

Index

'See-saw' movement, 157, **162**, 192
Sexually-transmitted diseases, 106
Sigmoid colon, 170. *See also* Intestinal tract
Sigmoid mesocolon, 170, 192-**193**
Sinusitis, 26
Skin, relation to liver, 104
Somatization of stress, 8
Sotto-Hall test. *See* Adson-Wright test
Sphincter of Oddi, 8. *See also* Bile ducts
    diagnosis, 136
    treatment, 91
Sphincter-like junctions, 7-8, 72, 192
Spleen
    anatomy, **152**-153
    function, 153
    palpation, 159
    pathology, 155-156
    treatment, 149, 151, 163
Splenic flexure, 182. *See also* Intestinal
    tract treatment, 186-187
Splenomegaly, 156
Stenosis, pyloric, 26, 80
Stomach
    anatomy, 71-72
    associated restrictions, 83-84
    diagnosis, 80-83
    diagnostic recoil, 82
    differential diagnosis, **80**-82
    function, 72-73
    inhibition points, 82
    pathology, 73-80
    prolapse. *See* Gastric prolapse
    strategy of treatment, 91-92
    therapeutic recoil, **86**-87

    treatment, 84-**87**, 88
Stool production, 173
Strategy for treatment, 24-25, 27
Subclavian artery, 14, 16
Surgery, 41, 57, 132

T

Thoracic outlet, 15
Toldt's fascia, 171, 189
Transverse colon, 170. *See also* Intestinal tract
Transverse mesocolon, **161**, 163, 170

U

Ulcer, 72, 74-75, 180
Ulcerative colitis, 179
Ultrasound, 26
Unwinding, 23, 24
Upledger, J., 23
Ureter, 207, 219-220
Ureteral calculi, 219-**220**
Uric acid, 104

V

Vomiting, 73-74

X

X-rays, 19-**20**, **21**